S0-DXD-131

Health and Healing

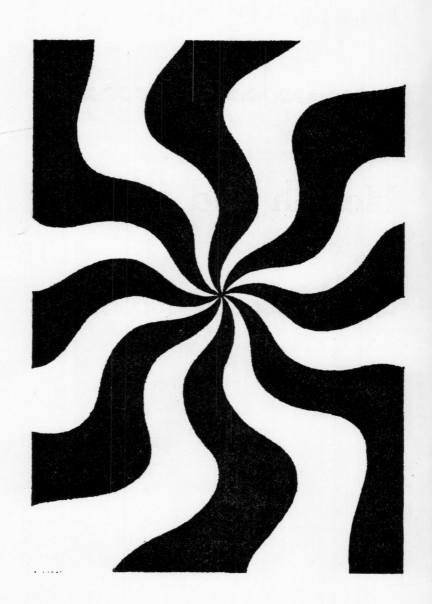

Health and Healing
by
Kaspar D. Naegele

&&&&&&&&&&&&&&&&&&&&&&&&&&&&&&&&&

Compiled and edited by

Elaine Cumming

Jossey-Bass Inc., Publishers

615 Montgomery Street · San Francisco · 1970

HEALTH AND HEALING
    By Kaspar D. Naegele
    Compiled and edited by Elaine Cumming

Library of Congress Catalog Card Number 73-110632

International Standard Book Number ISBN 0-87589-056-3

Manufactured in the United States of America
    Composed and printed by York Composition Company, Inc.
    Bound by Chas. H. Bohn & Co., Inc.

JACKET DESIGN BY WILLI BAUM, SAN FRANCISCO

FIRST EDITION

Code 7006

THE JOSSEY-BASS
BEHAVIORAL SCIENCE SERIES

General Editors

WILLIAM E. HENRY, *University of Chicago*

NEVITT SANFORD, *Wright Institute Berkeley*

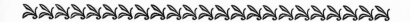

Foreword

The self-inflicted end of a life throws all that comes before into a debatable perspective. It would be difficult here to take the usual biographical road from "Kaspar Naegele was born as the first of three sons on February 16th, 1923, in Stuttgart; his father an artist, his mother a doctor . . . ," and proceed to schooling and degrees, marriage and three children, career, and the end. When the end is so disproportionately significant, one begins instead with: "Kaspar Naegele's life ended tragically in the Vancouver General Hos-

Foreword

pital on February 6th, 1965. He took it himself at the age of forty-two, after a long preoccupation with the subject of suicide both as a field of psychological and sociological inquiry and as a distinct option of personal conduct . . ."

But already words creep in that beg the question. His life ended "tragically," and suicide was an "option." In an age in which one may say with as much justification as a thousand years ago that "in the midst of life we are in death," the death of an individual becomes necessarily part of a context of collective suffering, and must be assimilated into the larger tragedy of an all-pervasive human condition characterized by the unceasing growth of the complexity of life and of the attendant strains on the psyche. In this context Kaspar Naegele's chosen "option" becomes easier rather than more difficult to accept, less shocking and more commensurate with contemporary life.

> *The courageous man starts to think no matter where he ends and no matter whether or not at that "end" . . . he can answer the nasty "so what?" Further, he raises disconcerting questions concerning Life and Death, without feeling that this is* ipso facto *a sign of perversion or weakness.*[1]

No doubt he very much lived his work. This is attested to not only by his extraordinary academic success and by his extensive bibliography, but also by the very themes he found to be legitimate subjects for scholarly inquiry: "The Necessity of Bedevilment," "Friendship and Acquaintances," "First and Further Thoughts on Sleep," and "The Sociology of Everyday Life." Although he remained in the academic sphere, his thinking and style of writing always pointing towards the

[1] All quotations are taken from the essay: "Student Freedom and Responsibility," originally read at the Fifth Canadian Hazen Conference in June, 1947, and reprinted in *The Dalhousie Review*, 1958, *28*, pp. 53–65.

Foreword

speculative and abstract, his work had also a clearly practical side. As Research Associate in Mental Health at the Harvard School of Public Health (1951–1953), as Lecturer for the School of Nursing at the University of British Columbia (1956–1958), as Chairman of the Scientific Planning Committee, British Columbia Branch, of the Canadian Mental Health Association (1957–1958), and as a member of the British Columbia Commission for Canadian Conference on Children (1958–1960), he found opportunities to apply his extraordinary sensitivities and uncanny appreciation of the complexities, ambivalences, and paradoxes in life to social betterment. All his work, inside and outside the classroom, was suffused by an intense personal commitment that accounts for the equally intense response and allegiance on the part of colleagues and students.

> *The degree of vitality needed in a university is of such a quality and quantity that one might well be justified in saying that both teacher and student should be possessed by a "daemon." A teacher or a student who is not possessed by a daemon is perverting his calling into a bureaucratic office in which he is easily replaced by one of a dozen other candidates.*

A distinction, therefore, between academic and applied sociology, or between the person and his intellectual pursuits, can be made only at the risk of missing the essence of Kaspar Naegele's nature.

One may point to his death as ultimate proof of a unity of thought and conduct, since he clearly saw and accepted the potential value and even the necessity of a self-imposed exit—an insight that transcended the vicissitudes of his own at times extremely troubled life. The intellectual roots of this insight lay far back in his youth and early thought:

> *Suffering—and somehow the whole area of suffering or tragedy, of the significance of death and so forth,*

*has been badly neglected in the systematic study of
man as it is now carried on through the social sciences—
refers to some of the effects of thinking and studying
on the scholar, and perhaps his audience. It may be
true that the truth shall make us free. It is, I think,
equally true that the process of discovery, certainly in
the social sciences, shall make us sad, at least for some
time.*

One may, however, describe his death as a result of a
failure of personality under stress, a failure whose roots could
also be traced far back, thus raising the possibility of alternative life courses that might have led to some more generally
acceptable conclusion. In so far as one accepts the idea of a
unity of thought and conduct, the suicidal end transcends
personal tragedy and becomes part of an intellectual profile. If
one accepts the idea of a life breaking under stress, one returns
to the thought of personal failure to survive in a life burdened
by work and responsibilities, a difficult childhood and adolescence, as well as domestic strains beyond the ordinary. No
doubt, a reading of these essays will allow an intellectual
profile to emerge that will make the first alternative more
persuasive. In that event some contribution to the understanding of suicide may inadvertently emerge—a consequence
quite in keeping with the concerns of a man who at the time of
his own death lectured on the very form it was to take.

Circumstances, as much as the complexion of his
mind, account for the fact that Kaspar Naegele lived his work.
The impressive academic path through McGill University
(B.A. 1945), Columbia University (M.A. 1947), and Harvard University (Ph.D. 1952), the long row of fellowships,
and the eventual progress from an instructorship in sociology at
the University of New Brunswick (1946–1947) to a deanship
at the University of British Columbia (1964) should not hide
the fact that his first professional choice would have been
medicine. Circumstances dictated the course of events, although

not always negatively: emigration from Germany (1937) to an English boarding school (Churchers College, Petersfield); internment as an enemy alien after Dunkirk and subsequent shipment under miserable conditions to Canada; release after eighteen months of detention—the result of administrative idiocy; admission to McGill with all hopes of medical studies dashed by financial impediments. What better vantage point for a future sociologist than to come from a mixed marriage, a product of the *Rassenschande* of pre-World War II Germany; to be deprived of family and home and sent to the kind of school bound to reinforce in a fifteen-year-old adolescent the sense of being an outsider; to voyage to Canada with German prisoners of war; to starve himself in order to convince the authorities to distinguish between military prisoners and refugees; to build a camp in Canada with compatriots under conditions challenging to the instinct for spiritual survival; to be at last released into the care of a businessman charged with, and overpaid for, the launching of a university career; to fight the immigration authorities for the right to study in the United States; to marry the daughter of a Canadian banker who looked upon his mongrel son-in-law with suspicion for what indeed he was—untypical, just too many unaccustomed things at once for comfort.

How productive for a sociologist to be a wanderer, an emigree, a perpetual visitor, to span the distance from the cow and horse-drawn wagons of a still dormant Swabian village between the wars to the expanse of the Pacific Far West. What better sources of insight than the menial labors in internment camps and work crews; the economically depressed academic beginnings in a New Brunswick shack without plumbing; the wide range of scholarly and social milieu that reached from the University of Oslo (1953–1954) to the Palo Alto Center for Advanced Studies in the Behavioral Sciences (1958–1959), and from provincial New Brunswick to cosmopolitan Cambridge, Massachusetts, and finally to a burgeoning University of British Columbia in Vancouver.

While the medical profession of Kaspar Naegele's mother was closed to him by circumstances, the artistic domains of father and brothers never ceased to influence him—to stir his impatience with the ultimate value of the Intellectual enterprise. None of his achievements—a classical German Gymnasium education, an Oxford-Cambridge Schools' Certificate with Distinction, a McGill B.A. with honors in sociology, a graduate education financed by prestigious fellowships, the encouragement and respect of teachers and colleagues, the final rise to the highest academic distinction—ever quite eradicated his nagging doubt of the value of the analytical vis-à-vis the creative intellect. Privately this doubt took shape as a sense of inferiority in relation to those in artistic pursuits. Intellectually it took the form of paradox.

> We have been witnessing the understandable and ironical fact that often much intellectual effort goes into discrediting the intellectual process. Marx and Freud are the most recent historical sources of this—which fact does not mean that both do not contribute indispensable and great sources of insight without which we would be very much blinder. Through the concepts of ideology and rationalization, much plausible contempt for the activity of thinking is set free. On further study, however, it would become clear that both terms contain considerable ambiguities. It would also become clear that we are involved in the inevitable circle within which we use reason and thought to discredit both. The schemes by which we have sought to demonstrate the irrationality of man have always been rational. Since these schemes also constitute part of man, there must be some significant limitations to his irrationality. It is clear that we need a new faith in the value of thinking and ideas . . .

A positive consequence of this perspective was his passionate demand to justify his work to himself through the personal impact of his teaching, and by bringing to bear on his teaching and writing the range of awareness, and the most far-roving interrelations and references in order to lend to his scholarship artistic freedom of form and creative élan.

> *We must restore our faith in intellectual activity by ridding that activity of some of its obvious sterility and fashioning it more after the activity of the artist. . . . We must conceive of teaching as an art, and of each lecture as an attempt at a work of art. . . . It is the nature of our ideas and information, the process of intellectual dialectic and style of our thought that should be our chief concern . . .*

A characteristic proviso follows immediately, however:

> *There seems to be an insoluble remnant to all problems. Worse still, one is driven to wonder whether all solutions must create further problems. . . . All, including those people committed to the intellectual life, seek for some kind of contentment. But probably the intellectual life, without which they would not be happy, needs as one of its preconditions, a productive level of discontent—with which they are also unhappy.*

If, indeed, the end of Kaspar Naegele's life does throw all its elements into a debatable perspective, then one may recognize in his perfectionism as a child and student, in his protracted battle to achieve self-esteem, in his unlimited academic perseverance, his deprivation of home through a lonely emigration, his adolescent idealism and innocence, in his sense of honor, his veneration of work, effort, and suffering, early ingredients contributing to a later tragedy—the tragedy of an unwillingness or inability to accept a certain kind of defeat or a flawed existence and self-image. However, may one not also arrange the life circumstances of this man, who loved to laugh and prized humor above everything, to understand the "end"

Foreword

as a resolution of a long-considered and ultimately lucid course of actions resulting from a lifelong effort to grasp the ramifications of self-assertion in family, profession, or society, and from a commitment to live his work. The moment of despair that precipitates the act is only the immediate cause. It occurs in the continuum of the preceding rational thought, ethical sophistication, and philosophical insight. The same ultimate act that can be seen as a failure under stress can become a logical and not altogether unacceptable or unredeemed consequence intimately related to the life and work it concludes.

> *The courageous man starts to think no matter where it ends. . . . He raises disconcerting questions concerning Life and Death, without feeling that this is* ipso facto *a sign of perversion or weakness.*

PHILIPP O. NAEGELE

Northampton, Massachusetts

Preface

It has been difficult to edit Kaspar Naegele's writing, for the text, like the man, is subtle and complex and no summaries are offered. Furthermore, although these essays were intended to form a book, they were left in varying degrees of completion. In preparing those that were still in draft, I was guided by notes in the margins of the manuscript, by the author's exchange of letters with colleagues, and by my own memory of this work.

These essays, like their author's speech, are full of the

interplay between opposing ideas. He loved paradox. Sometimes, just for the fun of it, he would include in one long sentence a complex statement and, parenthetically and playfully, its opposite. Because he knew that these Chinese-box constructions were hard to penetrate, I simplified some of them. Most of the verbal play that Kaspar Naegele loved has been left in. He enjoyed puns, play on words, and rhyming phrases. Once he called an essay on interdisciplinary research "Light Work or Spoiled Broth," a phrase containing parts of two maxims as well as a paradox. Occasionally, when the word play seemed to interrupt the meaning and I felt that I could have talked him out of it, I removed it.

Some of the details in these essays are out of date because they were written at the beginning of the 1960's, and the data on which they were based have been superseded. Nevertheless, the issues raised are as contemporary as if they had been thought out yesterday, and so no attempt has been made to bring the factual material up to date.

It has been my hope as I edited the less-finished parts of the essays that every sentence would speak in Kaspar Naegele's voice. Although I could often almost hear that voice, sometimes I may have missed his point. For any jarring notes I ask the forbearance of all who knew this wonderfully gifted man.

ELAINE CUMMING

Albany, New York
January, 1970

Contents

xix

Contents

Health and Healing

1

※※※※※※※※※※※※※※※※※※※※※※※※

Health and
Illness

✁✁✁✁✁✁✁✁✁✁✁✁✁✁✁✁✁✁✁✁✁✁✁✁

Why our concern with health? Why the persistence and growth of institutions and persons whose primary
interest is the well-being of others?

There is evidence enough that health is both a per-
vasive private concern and a persistent public issue: endless

advertisements remind us of remedies and precautions for
bodily and not-so-bodily conditions which in one way or
another are presumably symptoms of a less than healthy state.
In the name of public and private health we are urged to take
care of ourselves, to see doctors, to eat, to sleep, to work and
relax, to protect our teeth and watch our skin. We can hardly
watch a TV serial without seeing some member of the medical
profession at work. Indeed, the mass media encourage us, the
laity, to look at our medical professional resources, even though
they leave it deliberately unclear where fact and fiction meet
and diverge. Furthermore, if we have time and money, an
almost endless list of enterprises concerned with fighting various killers and enemies—from heart disease to cancer, from
madness to paralysis—awaits our cooperation. Finally, debates
over the right way of ordering our medical services in relation
to the public's good, the government's willingness, private
industry's interests, and the professions' demand for autonomy,
are conducted within hearing of us all. Thus, health is a public
topic, a public concern.

<h3 style="text-align:center">EXPERIENCE AND VALUE</h3>

The sources of our contemporary concern with illness
and health are several and arise in both our immediate experience and in our long-held values. Health, it would seem, is a
condition necessary for the realization of two of our regnant
values: mastery of the world, and fun. Illness impedes activity
and limits our autonomy. As such, it provides obstacles to an
activist philosophy that would bid us master the world. Illness
itself, therefore, becomes a matter of mastery; insofar as we
can, we reject a fatalistic view that would bid us to accept
external and internal events. Rather, illness is to be mastered,
prevented, cured, or limited. Being well, we are free to strive—
and to thrive. To thrive is indeed to be in full possession of
one's powers and to enjoy the play of these powers. Health

and fun, thus, come to be considered one of our rights, the more so when our lives are given meaning by on-going attempts at accomplishment. The "loss" of health, in other words, interferes. It interferes with what one wants to do, and interferes with what one wants to be. Interference, as a form of frustration and deprivation, must, in our society, be mastered and removed. Health is, therefore, both a condition of mastery and an object of it.

Pain, for all our Puritan heritage, is not a welcome experience. We do not cultivate it, except as an unavoidable accompaniment to learning and effort. We do not believe that pain, deliberately sought or inflicted, is a necessary condition for any specially valued experiences or attitudes; if it were, we would prefer to forgo them. Pain is to be reduced to a minimum, and the unavoidable minimum is to be only temporarily accepted. Pain, in other words, is seen as a limitation upon freedom and enjoyment, and although we may have to justify or accept such limitations in the form of punishment or as the result of our ignorance in the face of the forces of nature and of history, our desires tend toward the enhancement, in this life and on this earth, of our pleasures.

Illness is an enemy, inviting conquest. This conquest requires a number of things: knowledge and the organization necessary for the accumulation of knowledge, the application of knowledge through the work of professionally educated people, the division of labor necessary for this application and, finally, the marshaling of resources and the cultivation of attitudes that sustain the conquest. The wish for mastery and conquest of pain and deprivation automatically embeds the conquest in a far-flung web of institutions, and accordingly, the conquest of illness becomes a vested interest.

Health is also a vested interest, and as such it provides incomes, jobs, careers, and political issues. Health costs both the ill and the not-yet-ill money, and thus provides an income

3

for others. The economy of health—who should pay, when, how much, and to whom—is part of the wider economy of society as well as a special case for the ill member.

Why is the economy of health special? Because the costs of health radiate, affecting more than the individual, and because the costs of health are unpredictable and sometimes very high. Also, the economy of health is special because the consumer can be doubly helpless, for the plight from which he seeks escape requires outside aid. Illness provides one with an insufficiency, both of knowledge and of power. Even the well, because they are laymen, are relatively ignorant, and hence relatively helpless, in matters of body and soul. As consumers, therefore, the ill and the well are often not in a position to judge the service and product that they are given. We believe in the mastery of illness by rational means, and our health becomes the concern of a specialized minority. Thus our concern with health is at once an expression of our wish for autonomy and freedom from fateful resignation, and, at the same time, a source of dependence.

Illness, by and large, happens to us—to any of us, although we differ in our chances for contracting different kinds of illness. Our inequalities, furthermore, give our illnesses rather different consequences, even though in the most general sense we are equal in our capacity for becoming incapacitated. Our concern with health, furthermore, provides us with an opportunity for seeking part of the equality to which North American culture tends to be committed. Health, like literacy, has a double face in this respect: it is part of the condition of participation in social life, but it is also an accomplished state that, in the name of various ideals, including justice and efficiency, should be within the reach of all. Health thus provides an opportunity for the exercise of democratic beliefs, and exercising these beliefs leads, in turn, to the establishment of an inclusive set of institutions.

4

Health and Illness

Health as a valued state is increasingly considered a right that should be realized regardless of the inequalities of history and society. It is a right to which we all have a claim, regardless of our ability to pay for it. Because of our inescapable social involvement, health for any one of us is contingent upon the health of many others, because illness is contagious in more than one sense. The enjoyment of health is impossible as a radically autonomous venture, unaffected by the health of others; yet as the claim for equality of health becomes more firmly established, the debate over implementing this claim becomes sharper. Thus health as a social issue presents an opportunity for debate about many things that give meaning and direction to our society.

Concern with health is part of a wider pattern of intellectual and moral development. The extension of science, the systematic charting of natural conditions, social arrangements, and particularly inner dispositions have demonstrated the nonrational, sensuous, and aesthetically appreciative desires and capacities of human beings. Our concern with health is thus part of our wider concern with and greater attention to the passions, including the passions of sexuality. The fate of the passions in a modern urban world becomes a matter of a special attention that is part of the enhanced self-consciousness characteristic of modern societies.

High standards of health, low rates of infant mortality, and increased longevity are the measures, as well as the ingredients, of high standards of living. Such standards refer not only to the comparative lot of many people, but they also allow comparison between nations. Because of these comparisons, health becomes a measure of both advantage and accomplishment, making for invidious comparison between and within societies. Concerns about health become woven into both ideological and concrete struggles.

Cleanliness, saneness, and wholeness of body and mind

5

are valued assets and are enjoyed in their own right; what is healthy and what is desirable come to be equated. The commitment to health as a general value, and the investment of large resources of time and money in it, suggests, for appraisal, the following further considerations:

In North America, the concern with health exists in four domains: first, health is a professional responsibility and, as such, the object of scientific inquiry; second, health is a political and legislative matter; third, health provides purposes for many voluntary as well as lay organizations; and finally, health is inevitably a private and personal concern. The plethora of voluntary efforts and agencies dealing with health suggests, however, that the concern with health feeds on a richer compound of public and private motives than those suggested in the previous pages.

Three motives for this concern with health stand out: first, we wish to maintain our liberty while maintaining health, and such liberty demands freedom in the choice of doctors, confidentiality in our dealings with those who professionally aid us in our plight, and the right to keep our medical histories private. The concern with health, in other words, is always intertwined with other concerns. Second, our interest in health thrives on fear and anxiety, although sometimes these feelings are created less by ourselves and more by others. Whatever their source, fear and anxiety contribute to our willingness to participate in various specific routines, from personal hygiene to regular medical examinations. Participation in organized voluntary activities can also take its impetus from such fears and the more so when they are associated with sentiments of philanthropy. Third, when all these motives and forces converge, health becomes established as a vested interest linking private needs with public values and arrangements. As a value, health has features that give it a special place in the company of the general values by which we live. That company includes

6

the belief in mastery, in equality, in individual scope, and in security, although one can, even to a large degree, reject such values; one can cultivate in their stead mystic otherworldliness, passivity, a belief in the hierarchical ordering of social life, or a radical commitment to free enterprise and competition.

Health as a value cannot be similarly rejected. To be radically opposed to it is to invite death. Short of such radicalism, however, there is still much scope for opposition. One can reject the medical domain in the name of various commitments either to nature, religion, or cultural forms distant in place or time. One can be a Christian Scientist or a vegetarian, an ardent opponent of fluoridation or a new-won disciple of acupuncture. One can, thus, choose to oppose either the specific methods of the day or the general emphasis given to health. One can seek to ignore health, perhaps precisely because one believes that health, including sanity, flourishes best when least watched. One can instead, perhaps for rather similar reasons, make much too much of health. One can, finally, upset the balance that governs the official philosophy of health embodied in our society.

This balance derives from trying to make our peace among at least three general inclinations. Two of these have been named the traditions of Hygeia and of Asclepius, the one standing for the preventive virtues of a sane life, wisdom, and sensible conduct, and the other standing less for prevention and more for restitution. Asclepius represented competent mastery of the accidents of life. Health, in the name of these rival ideals, is thus at once a matter of sane living within the natural order of things and a matter of the deliberate restitutive treatment of nature mismanaged. This opposition of tradition includes a number of contrasts. First, a belief in wise living as a means to health suggests a belief in the fundamental harmony of nature, and even a belief that medicine can disclose natural laws. Such a belief assumes that men, guided by this disclosure, will follow these laws, and will find this to their advantage. Asclepius was more pessimistic, or more realistic, than Hygeia. His cult suggests that whether nature be fundamentally harmonious or not, men are more than sensible, and they are also driven by various desires. The prevention of illness and accident or the enhancement of health are not man's only end.

The cultivation of health, in the end, comes to be a compromise between Hygeia and Asclepius; beyond that, it becomes a compromise between these two emphases and a third general inclination, a concern with supernatural realms that differ both from those of nature and from those of men. Although the religious traditions of our society are too various to have a single and specific relation to health as an ideal or condition of life on earth, and doctrinal formulations are not necessarily the major way in which a religious tradition becomes associated with matters of illness and health, the general religious preference of our society nevertheless reinforces the kind of "activism" that provides illness with the salience we afford it. Furthermore, as illness comes to be genuinely considered an attribute of a person as a whole, the religious and the medical domains become simultaneously new colleagues and new competitors. With few exceptions, however, the religious domain neither seeks illness nor cultivates an indifference toward it, but is sympathetic toward the conquest of illness, and subscribes to the fight against pain and deprivation.

Finally, health as a desired end is both ubiquitous and empty. One is never without it, but it is never clear what precisely one possesses in having it. To be sure, we can point to specific experiences when we describe ourselves as enjoying good health or suffering ill health, but these are imprecise; a very large range of states are ascribed to good or ill health. States of good health may be an end in themselves, being potentially a source of satisfaction, but such satisfaction derives from the sense of well-being, which, in turn, thrives on more than the absence of pain. On the other hand, pain can drive all other desires away, except the desire to be free of it. In this way pain need be no further defined: it is to be avoided, reduced, conquered. But freedom from it only clears the decks, and what is to occupy these decks when they are cleared? A healthy mode of existence? That stands for more than it says, for it implies answers to diverse questions. Today these questions are subject to continuous debate, to contrary answers. Accordingly, the emphasis on some kinds of positive health, about which at first glance we might all agree, is in part a solution to an embarrassment—how can one be against it—unless one can define precisely what one means by it?

Ultimately, it becomes apparent that health is only one more name for a pattern of values that mark what we loosely call the middle class. Health, undefined, is usefully vague; as such, it is potentially a focus for general moral agreement, even for many specific undertakings for which people are more or less willing to volunteer. Because of its vagueness, rather than despite it, health can be one of those general moral goods to which otherwise disagreeing individuals and groups can collectively subscribe.

SOME PUBLIC FACTS

Daily, quarterly, and annually, diverse agencies, both public and private, publish a host of information on many aspects of the fact that men fall ill. These figures, suspended between statistical accounts of births and deaths, constitute a growing, increasingly worldwide (if not world-uniform) accounting system of how many are ill, how often, in what manner, and at what cost. Inevitably these figures have come to include numerical accounts of the characteristics of the

9

healing professions and institutions. The following is a cursory reference to one such attempt to tame the divergent facts that issue from human illness.

In 1951, under the auspices of the United Nations, the International Labor Office, and the World Health Organization, a "Report on the World Social Situation"[1] was issued. The very existence of such a report is a remarkable evidence of man's attempt to extend the mastery of the world to include social patterns and individual lives. We cannot, here, concern ourselves with the adequacy of the various reporting systems, usually sustained by national governments, from which such generalizations must be drawn, but these facts seem worth considering:

All over the world success in improving the physical conditions of health has been growing. More people live longer.

There are still large differences between countries in mortality from infectious and parasitic diseases. One stands a much better chance to die from one of these diseases in, say, Colombia than in Holland. Still, rapid progress has been made everywhere in the reduction of mass diseases such as malaria. The countries known as "developing," in which, until recently, communicable diseases were still uncontrolled, have shown the most dramatic improvements, whereas in developed areas past success now confronts more recalcitrant obstacles. In the more industrialized countries, degenerative diseases, heart ailments, senility, and cancer constitute the major source of physical plight demanding professional management and successful prevention. There has been, for instance, an increase in the incidence of certain forms of cancer, especially cancer of the respiratory system, whereas other forms, such as cancer of the digestive organs, have increased more slowly but

[1] *Report on the World Social Situation.* New York: United Nations, 1957, especially Chapter 3, pp. 28–48.

10

"still appear to take more lives than any other type of malignancy." We should add, too, that in modern societies, "as in the case of mortality from cancer of the respiratory organs, mortality from cancer of the digestive organs is higher . . . among men than women."[2]

There has been a constant increase in the incidence of accidents. Such accidents involve machines, especially transport facilities.[3] There again, the death ratio, according to the United Nations Report, is much higher among men than among women.[4]

With increasing worldwide industrialization, the problems of environmental sanitation that face the less-developed countries are being solved and displaced by new hazards. The latter derive from problems associated with the supervision of water supplies, sewage collection and disposal, the management of diverse kinds of industrial waste, and the control of artificial radiation.

Concern with mental illness, even if only measured by the numbers of all hospital beds occupied by people with a diagnosis of some kind of emotional disturbance, is becoming more widespread throughout the world. Professional resources and institutional facilities devoted to the management of emotional plights are increasing.

Countries differ considerably in the ratios of physicians, nurses, and hospital beds to populations. In India, for instance, in 1950 there was one hospital bed for every 3,060 inhabitants. In Scotland at that time, the ratio was one bed to 98 inhabitants. In Africa, with a population of about 211 million, there were sixteen medical schools, and about 9,000

[2] *Report on the World* . . . , p. 38.
[3] For a thought-stimulating, though cautiously to be interpreted research report, see A. L. Porterfield, "Traffic Fatalities, Suicide and Homicide," *American Sociological Review*, 1960, *25* (6), pp. 897–901.
[4] Porterfield, p. 38.

patients per physician. In Europe, with a population of 619 million, there were 253 medical schools and 931 patients for each doctor.[5] Such figures need careful interpretation, since ratios of this kind leave one quite uninstructed about the actual distribution of health services, including doctors, in a given country, or about the use people make of what is available to them. Besides, to a certain degree, "objective facts" are surrounded by various subjective assumptions and beliefs; in modern societies, as in others, just as some still prefer to hide their money in socks rather than entrust it to banks, others prefer home remedies to professional encounters.

The unequivocal facts of physical condition and the more elusive facts of emotional plight, are, then, unequally distributed within and between societies, and both have social consequences; in complicated and unequal ways they also have social roots. Measurable illness, like cancer, occurs with unequal frequency at different stages of the life-cycle or at unequal rates to men and women. Indeed, in modern societies, men tend in general to have more illnesses and shorter lives than women. None of these differences by age and stage is entirely biological in origin.

A considerable widening of the concept of health itself has accompanied changing rates of illness. Many countries are now involved in the discussion and planning of comprehensive health services while at the same time experimenting with the development of local health units. Such units, as well as those private cooperative arrangements that involve the coordination of various specialist services, seek to combine the advantages of specialization with an acceptance of the fact that each individual case is a unique person who contributes to wider patterns that will survive him.

The study of rates of different kinds of plight has

[5] Porterfield, pp. 45–48.

contributed both to the management of individual plights and to the understanding of society. Management and understanding together yield some general ideas:

There is no one theory of the cause of any and all illness, the more so since illness as a term refers alike to influenza and ulcers, alcoholism and meningitis, nephritis and schizophrenia. Accordingly, the curative domain, like society itself, must be hospitable in its thought and practice to the management of several causal orders, organic and psychological, symbolically shared and institutional. This hospitality in turn creates complexity in the curative domain, prolongs professional education, and invites controversy. Such controversy involves debate about the relative importance of the several causal orders, and the controversy is kept alive by the intellectual and practical demand for an economy in our conception, and hence management, of illness. Such demand for economy is one of the roots of orthodoxy. The curative domain is thus torn between complexity and simplicity, suspended between the wish to be just to the theoretical puzzles of illnesses and the wish to keep manageable its practical healing obligations. Those, such as chiropractors, who are considered to be solving their problems with oversimplicity are set apart and kept at the circumference of the professional curative domain.

Satisfactory explanations of the prevalence and incidence of such countable plights as alcoholism, ulcers, cancer, and emotional disturbance must always lead to an understanding of the individual case. The reverse, however, is not true. Just as deep immersion in individual biographies considered one at a time cannot be counted upon to lead to an understanding of such transcendent matters as ideology, the endemic strains of social organization, or the preventive by-products of religious rituals, so the study of individual cases fails to explain their prevalence.

Health and Healing

Attempts to account for variations in the rates of suicide and alcoholism illustrate concretely the gradient from social cause to individual effect. In both cases, socially distinct categories such as men and women, socially supported and socially isolated individuals, and morally guided and morally aimless persons differ in their susceptibility to these two forms of escaping from the daily world.[6] The low rate of alcoholism among Jews, for example, has been consistently observed. Typically, the nonalcoholic Jew is not an abstainer. Rather, he has learned to drink as a child from familiar adults in the context of religious and social ritual. He drinks, in part at least, to worship, and thus learns to contain his consumption within the boundaries compatible with maintaining a relaxed and sensible sobriety.[7] Such an explanation falls far short, however, of suggesting a reason for the high rate of alcoholism among men of Irish descent.[8] The alcoholic sometimes seems to rebel against an abstaining past, learns to drink in the context of a rebellious adolescence from peers who are similarly driven, or perhaps he learns from compulsively drinking parents. In using drinking as a means to various ends, he acts out rebellion and passivity in a progressively more expensive and physically debilitating pattern.[9] A whole array of forces, childhood and religious tradition, inner drives, and the physiological properties of both men and alcohol converge in the explanation of

[6] See, for instance, A. F. Henry and J. F. Short, Jr., *Suicide and Homicide*. Glencoe, Ill.: Free Press, 1954. Also, R. G. McCarthy, *Drinking and Intoxication*. Glencoe, Ill.: Free Press, 1959.

[7] C. R. Snyder, *Alcohol and the Jews, a Cultural Study of Drinking and Sobriety*. Glencoe, Ill.: Free Press, 1958.

[8] D. D. Glad, "Attitudes and Experiences of American-Jewish and American-Irish Male Youth as Related to Differences in Adult Rates of Inebriety," *Quarterly Journal of Studies on Alcohol*, 1947 8(3), pp. 406–472.

[9] See R. G. McCarthy, *Drinking and Intoxication*. Glencoe, Ill.: Free Press, 1959, pp. 263–277.

why some who drink become alcoholic and others much like them do not.

Society touches on our illnesses at least at three points: in their genesis, in their unfolding history, and in their consequences. In practice, we have been least successful in establishing in a reliable fashion, the social genesis and individual motives of our illnesses. When we look back, we are often too late in our attempts to understand causation and must confine ourselves to reconstructing the past from present accounts; when we look forward, we do not feel free to let an ominous present automatically predict a pathological future.

Given social causation, still we can see that social arrangements inevitably involve individual biographies. All social arrangements involve a combination of demands and rewards, and individuals can be viewed in turn as a configuration of resources and liabilities, variously able to be their own masters and to respond to the regnant demands of others. Between social arrangements on the one hand and the resources and liabilities of individuals on the other, there exist certain classic strains; these include contradictory demands, unclear expectations, obligations unmatched by the requisite resources, unrealizable standards, excessive diversity or constraint, and inadequate provisions for a productive balance of coherence and autonomy. Yet the formulation of these social strains, which are in themselves causes of some of our plights, relies both on a view of individual biography and on certain general values. In the end it is probably not possible to separate what is necessary from what is desirable when one comes to formulate patterns of individual life histories. To put it differently: our plights occur within history relative to certain shared values and certain schemes of social organization. If, for example, we are concerned with alcoholism, whether our concern is with the magnitude of the overall problem or with the individual case, our explanations must sooner or later include notions of the meaning of this illness—meaning to those who are ill and to those to whom the ill are significant. Its meaning, presumably, includes a poignant exchange of one kind of restraint for another: Freedom from certain pains is bartered for freedom from dependence on an impersonal master. To put it this way, requires notions of freedom. Such notions are constituted in the moral discourse of our particular culture.

The history and management of diseases necessarily involve other people. Thus, whatever its source, illness is inescapably social, and it is never more obviously so than when the attempt to cure consists in removing the patient from society. Such a decision is usually made by, or in collaboration with, some member of the healing professions.

MEDICINE AS A PROFESSION

Industrialized societies, as we have come to know and to need them, would be impossible without the professions, which constitute a mode of work typically involving fairly direct relations to clients, and which at the same time demand a recognition of the difference between themselves and the laity.

The professions provide services that require specialized knowledge and competence. They represent a form of mastery by the few over problems that can in principle afflict the many. As a rule, professional knowledge and competence are required by the uninitiated from already established professional persons. The latter, through a series of complicated organizations, provide for their own replacement and determine the processes of selection that govern access to the ranks of the profession. Today, the professions are typically a kind of monopoly that remains assigned to them as long as each profession is able to provide and license enough practitioners to meet the demand for their service.

Professions are called upon to apply the knowledge

they have, and application always transcends knowledge; it involves skill, guess, and risk. Application involves, in other words, the exercise of judgment and the assumption of responsibility. Professions are governed by relatively explicit bodies of moral tradition, usually called professional ethics, by which the members both reassure those dependent on them of their good intentions and facilitate the cooperation and obedience necessary for the successful enactment of professional responsibilities. Clearly, professions differ in these matters. Librarians, for instance, unlike doctors, are not involved in matters of life and death, although, like doctors, they may be called upon to make judgments of considerable consequence, such as withholding or suggesting reading matter that has a fairly direct bearing on the experience of the reader. Most of the professions, however, and especially law, medicine, engineering, and the clerical profession, are alike in being full-time occupations, and their members make a career of their professional work.

In a certain sense all the professions, but medicine especially, stand apart as communities within communities.[10] They generate a sense of colleagueship to buttress their difference from the laity. They seek the qualities of the ordinary man undiluted by the ordinary weakness. They combine attachment to a gentlemanly tradition, with its emphasis on learning, to a steadiness in judgment and demeanor, with its emphasis on scientific, technical, and specialized competence, acquired during a long and standardized training.

Typically, the professions sustain relations to specific clients, to whom they are expected to give of themselves. The professional is expected to combine generalized knowledge with particular treatment, yet use imaginative procedures that are at the same time steadfast, and lacking in the kind of erratic

[10] See W. J. Goode, "Community Within a Community: The Professions," *American Sociological Review,* 1957, 22(2), pp. 194–200.

ups and downs that are sometimes associated with the creative arts. (Nevertheless, we refer to *professional artists* and the *healing arts*.)

Healing, in our society, tends toward professional practice. It looks back on a long, if uneven, professional history, and has its own classical heroes. But medicine must continue its tradition under circumstances that are very different from its origins; its professional position, moreover, contains a series of potentially quite contrary elements from which some kind of balance must be forged; these elements include: concern for the immediate demands of patients versus a commitment to continuous self-education; attachment to the humble skepticism that accompanies scientific inquiry versus the willingness to assume risks and take action; enhancement of specialized competence versus the adherence to a well-rounded and cultivated style of living; attachment to those forces that improve man's lot versus the cultivation of the spirit of neutrality that suspends moral judgment of the individual conduct; a just concern with the plight of any and all patients versus the unavoidable necessity to earn a living and so to consider the patient's ability to pay; and a dominating concern for the welfare of others versus the right to have a normal and private life of one's own.

These tensions reflect the relationship of the practice of medicine to both the patients who come for help and the corporate medical body. In short, the practicing physician is attached to two poles, his constituents and his colleagues.

HEALING AS A CALLING

Except in the case of married women, we expect doctors to give their full-time attention to the pursuit of medicine. Admittedly, they may pursue medicine in a variety of forms other than practicing it. They may do research, or teach, or administer, or work in a bureaucratic setting such as public health. Still, within broad limits, we expect them to be readily available to their patients, and even to allow intrusions into their private lives, justified by the unpredictable character of medical emergencies; neither babies nor fractures, nor acute infections or heart attacks respect office routines. But we know that there are many subtle and direct ways by which doctors educate their patients to confine their demands to a definite time schedule. Some doctors have learned how to spare themselves in such ways as by deflecting night calls to younger colleagues. Ultimately, however, we expect medicine to be a full-time occupation and to remain a man's job throughout his lifetime. Having regulated entry into medicine, the profession expects no losses from it except by death. These attitudes help establish the autonomy of the medical profession and to limit those conflicts that would arise were medical activities combined with other prominent occupational, political, or religious functions.

In practice, of course, the matter is considerably more complicated than our ideals would lead us to believe, but certain things are clear: we do not expect, for instance, a justice in the Supreme Court of the United States to have previously practiced medicine. Nor is it any longer possible, except in a very few instances, to combine civic and medical accomplishments in the fashion of a Benjamin Rush. Today, professionalization and specialization do not permit one man such an array of accomplishments, although the connection between medicine as a professional activity and the scholarly pursuit of the humanistic traditions (a connection relevant to the cultivation of competence) has become a subject of continuous concern and argument. Medical education, as well as medical practice, is a full-time and specialized occupation, but at the same time we are in the midst of many experiments to reintroduce more flexibility and more humanistic pursuits into the medical curriculum.

Health and Healing

We do not know at the moment the precise patterns that govern the participation by doctors, as doctors, in those domains of society that are not themselves directly connected with medicine. We do know, on the one hand, that professional autonomy is in large measure tantamount to professional neutrality in the face of the cleavages and controversies that mark a complicated society. On the other hand, however, we know that the special interests of religion, ethnicity, and labor unions all help to create institutions, such as hospitals, that associate the medical profession with some of the major recognizable segments of society. Still, we expect physicians and nurses alike to refrain from using their professional intimacy with the inner lives of their patients for purposes of religious or political influence or conversion. We know, of course, that by extension of the notion of colleagueship, doctors, nurses, and various more specialized medical or quasi-medical groups constitute themselves into regional and national corporate organizations whose activities are by no means confined to clinical endeavors.

As a rule, such bodies have a double face. On the one hand, they are forums for the exchange of technical knowledge concerning the substance of a profession's work; and on the other, they are guardians or representatives of the emergent interests of a profession. They are concerned with its status, conditions of work, remuneration, and connection with society. We know that the American Medical Association, for instance, undertakes an extensive set of activities to forestall what it calls undue governmental interference or the establishment of so-called socialized medicine. We know, too, that membership in professional corporate organizations is virtually a constituent of professional life. Such membership helps to establish the notion of colleagueship by giving it external and visible form; it provides for mutual solidarity in the face of a laity that

20

cannot help having a distorted view of those helpers on whom it depends, yet whom it also must pay.

The support of corporate professional groups can, in many instances, also work to restrain and limit the expression of private preferences, even when they are compatible with the main professional tradition. We further know that such large, voluntary organizations as the British and American Medical Associations are subject to the general problems of large organizations. They manifest tendencies toward oligarchy and concern with efficiency. We are aware, for example, that in the United States urban physicians and specialists stand a better chance for political office in the American Medical Association than rural or general practitioners. Moreover, membership in professional organizations is usually a necessary condition for hospital appointment. Also, these societies have power to punish serious medical offenses; sometimes such offenses involve practices that arouse the jealousy of colleagues rather than causing damage to patients. Finally, the American Medical Association, in general, and county societies in particular, help to set educational standards, whereas state societies tend to dominate licensing boards, influence the development of various health insurance plans, and tend, through journals and other publications, to formulate and disseminate a tradition of opinion from which dissent is not always possible.

A just view of all these matters is not easy. We are dealing with a situation of competing interests that include the legitimate rights of individual practitioners, the rights of individual patients, the requirements of corporate organizations to maintain tradition and colleagueship, and the social requirements for equal and effective medical care. All of these interests are potentially in conflict; they certainly do not represent a predetermined natural harmony.

Medical organizations, like all human organizations,

Health and Healing

are subject to change. An American Medical Association approves today what it may have viewed with concern and disapproval ten or twenty years ago. It was unable to prevent the growth of group practice and health plans that in the early stages it viewed with displeasure; a series of legal battles further advanced these developments. In England, the British Medical Association has become a powerful partner in the national health scheme that in many respects it clearly helped to institute and arrange. It is a moot question whether, besides being pressure groups, national medical associations are also explicit political forces within the terms of party politics. Clearly, a professional organization will refrain from formally endorsing a political party, because this would contradict its avowed tradition of neutrality, and it would lose those opportunities for cure and mediation that it derives precisely from being an understanding refuge in a punitive world.

Under certain conditions, the organization of medicine becomes especially important. Dutch doctors under the German occupation, for instance, organized themselves against collaboration with the labor draft by assisting with the medical selection of labor deportees. This organization helped physicians not to betray their professional secrets and not to report persons with wounds; it protested in 1944 and 1945 against the food conditions in Holland and it "confronted the German administration with the responsibility for the general decline of good public health."[11]

We expect doctors to become wholly part of the medical domain while allowing them a private life. We expect them also to be part of a generally educated sector of the community and, as such, to be more than technicians. We expect them, finally, to be colleagues one to another.

[11] W. Warmbrunn, *The Netherlands Under the German Occupation, 1940–1945.* Unpublished doctoral dissertation, Stanford, May 1955, p. 237.

Health and Illness

Recently, changes in the status of women and changes in the age of marriage have produced some new exceptions to the pattern of a lifetime commitment to professional healing. It is now possible for married women in medicine and, even more so in nursing, to leave their work for varying periods of time and to return when children are older, husbands are willing, or their own inclinations have revived. Such withdrawal and return further stimulates the insistence on continuing education that is becoming established within professional life.

2

Body, Mind, and Pain

We are born, we work, talk, sleep, and die. We are obviously embodied creatures, yet we apprehend this fact with the help of ideas and representations. Even though the organism is necessary for experience, and the brain is necessary for thought, experience and thought nevertheless represent an orderliness and a succession of associations of their own, apart from body and brain.

BODY AS A SOCIAL PHENOMENON

The puzzling relationship between mind and matter has been the occasion for a huge amount of debate, dogma, and thought. All the controversies among different philosophies, different religious views concerning ultimate reality, as well as the scientific debates about the relative autonomy or mutual reducibility of the social and natural sciences and their various subdivisions, are dramatic and interesting, although sometimes wearisome, and all of them we must leave to one side.

However, we cannot omit some summary references to human embodiedness itself. It is as a host to illness that our bodies become the subject of medical intervention. Such intervention is, however, only one of several kinds of intervention to which our bodies are subject. We paint ourselves, dress ourselves, and shape ourselves with some reference to a succession of fashions. In some societies we even bind feet or breasts, or try to affect the shape of our heads.

Several varied and complicated facts about the body can be condensed into a few simple observations:

First, the ground plan of the human body is a relatively constant one. As such it stands in interesting contrast to the changing history and structure of human societies, which, though changing, consistently depend on the embodiedness of the populations that constitute them. Indeed, if we wish to quell our sense of the curious intangibility of social arrangements by giving them definite substance, we speak of the incorporation of this or that association, township, or economic concern, which helps us to feel that, like us, these arrangements have identity and boundaries. Its apparent separateness is one of the human body's outstanding features.

25

Health and Healing

Second, illness can be one avenue to death; so can accidents, suicide, or murder. The possibility of death gives us our sharp sense of corporeal coherence. In death the body's coherence is dissolved in irreversible fashion.

Third, we experience our bodies at the same time that we constitute images of them. The experience and image of the body depend on many of the properties of the body itself. One of these, important for human society, is the capacity of the human body to coordinate its activities with those of others. To a degree this coordination requires self-consciousness; obversely, all life in society leads to an image of oneself. The self, as has been implicit throughout, is a social phenomenon. It can arise only when, at the beginning of our life-cycle, we are in the presence of others on whom we depend for survival and whose conception of themselves and of us we learn to make part of ourselves. Thus, our body becomes a possession of a self that arises through our relations to others. These others treat us in their image; their image includes a notion of ourselves and of themselves.[1]

Fourth, the images we have of our bodies may be quietly kept to ourselves, but they are dependent on the values about the body held in circles whose judgments, one way or another, we value or fear. This is particularly obvious with regard to such familiar phenomena as age and sex. Clearly age and sex are physical facts, but they are no more so than all other social facts. For our purposes, age and sex, as different attributes of the human body, are also important aspects of the organization of social relations.

Fifth, the fact that the human organism comes in two major classes, male and female, obviously affects social arrangements deeply. A society able to survive through the asexual

[1] These thoughts find a classical exposition in the work of G. H. Mead, *Mind, Self, and Society*. Chicago, Ill.: University of Chicago Press, 1934.

26

mechanisms of parthenogenesis would be unimaginably different. Similarly, the organic facts of male and female bodies are inextricably elaborated by the social meanings that we learn to give this natural contrast. The character of the biochemical and anatomical contrast in itself helps to set limits and give direction to the varieties of social agreements by which this contrast is further elaborated and exaggerated, and sometimes minimized. The social import of "male" and "female" finally comes to stand in anything but a simple relation to the so-called givens of nature.[2] All this is obvious, and yet easily forgotten, especially since the continuities of nature are often obscured by the radical distinctions of society.

The division between male and female is, as we also know, a learned accomplishment despite its origin in biological resources and requirements. It is, moreover, almost always an irrevocable difference as well as a nontransgressible one. We must *be* men or women, and we can only be one or the other. By contrast, we move through our age, as we exchange one stage in a life span for another.

Sixth, the differentiation of the human body—into male and female, old and young—helps to introduce that "severalness" that always characterizes human arrangements. This severalness is both expressed and produced by the fact that society, even in its simplest forms, always involves a division of labor and an allocation of power and responsibility. These divisions and allocations, in turn, offer the resources of the body unequal chances of further development, be it in the form of growth or in the form of illness.

Seventh, time binds into one familiar web the experience of the body as a maturing and declining organism. In the West we tend to think of life as a finite stream of events

[2] Cf. E. Fromm, "Sex and Character," in R. Anshen (Ed.), *The Family: Its Function and Destiny.* New York: Harper and Brothers, 1949, pp. 375–392.

27

suspended between two radical occurrences, birth and death. Illness, too, is a course of events; but in addition it marks a coincidence of partly antithetical orders—human organisms and micro-organisms. When illness takes the form of emotional disturbance, on the other hand, disturbances in the very history of the individuals who are ill become the focus of attention.

Eighth, the body is an object of social regulation and evaluation. Through the patterns surrounding age and sex, we gain our identities, establish ourselves in intimate and distant circles, regulate under what conditions we may share what intimacies with whom, and so generate not only a complicated sense of what is appropriate, but also a sense of the difference between the private and the public. In substance, these matters are anything but universal, but in form, the distinctions between private and public and between the self and the other are longstanding and widespread aspects of human living.

Ninth, notions of integrity and sacredness adhere to the body. In Western society we have gone very far in forbidding such deliberate manipulations as binding of breasts or feet, the elongation of the head, the splitting of lips, or the kind of superincisions still found in certain nonliterate societies. Still, we do not leave the body "as it is." Different social circles prefer different shapes and weights, and, with a deliberate use of diet, we more or less successfully produce desired or desirable figures. Moreover, we allow the sexes very different privileges in this regard. We expect women, except in a few circles, to have their lips painted by the time they emerge as potential lovers or mothers. We expect most men to be shaved and to wear their hair short. Variations in these matters become attached to other distinctions and thus help constitute those differences in social status or styles of life or self-conception that, for one reason or another, our various traditions require.

28

Body, Mind, and Pain

Tenth, since we live within the basic intangibleness of social arrangements and mutual expectations, the concrete singularity of the body is a welcome opportunity for expressing here and now many subtle notions.

The ground plan of the body provides opportunity for the experience of our particular singularity and for the elaboration of certain ideas of privacy. It also provides us with the experience that we are intimately connected, as self-conscious creatures, to an organic structure that is never free from the alternation of pleasure and pain. On the very well-being of the body, in turn, depend at least certain experiences and accomplishments. Unaided, we can know fairly little about the body; yet to invade it in any systematic manner would evoke pain. Indeed, a literal insight into the body is quite intolerable for many to whom the sight of blood, quite apart from the shock of injury, provides but an exercise of their sense of fear or disgust. The strangeness of the body thus provides interesting balances for the sense of intimacy that we also develop toward it. Only the individual can fully know his own pain or pleasure.

The facts condensed in these ten points are quite differently acknowledged, or hidden, by members of different circles. Besides, the radical distinction between the body as a physical order and the body as a possession by and of the self is impossible to maintain for long. Furthermore, the medical profession, as an established enterprise, must cultivate a steady sense of the body as an impersonal and physical order, and medical scientists have to believe that the detailed structure and processes of the body are progressively knowable. This view helps to set the medical profession apart from the rest of us, even from those who pride themselves on their rationality or their equanimity in the face of such crises of the body as injury or death. Only deliberate training and experience provide this access to the "inside" of the body. Actually the body

29

finally becomes the scene of great and rapidly growing knowledge precisely when such nonvisible features as the functions of the blood become technically and intellectually visible.

Because mass communication thrives on the general interest in the inner mysteries that our skins surround, much specialized knowledge concerning the body has ceased to be esoteric, although a large part of our knowledge is still a matter of professional monopoly. Public libraries tend to have specific rules governing the loaning of medical textbooks, when they own them at all. Operations, however, are now televised so that we can see the heartbeats of strangers. In addition, contemporary attitudes toward sexuality have strengthened the forces that would reduce the hiddenness of the body from view, discussion, or inspection. The incidence of all these developments is varied, both between Western societies and within them. Nakedness is unequally cultivated by different groups within the same population. To some, especially Roman Catholics, the sacred givenness of the body, even when dead, retains its demand for a respect that excludes cremation as a legitimate way of disposing of it.

We do not know too much about the value that different circles of our society place upon the body, nor do we have any systematic information concerning the image that is held of the body. We know that body images tend to be distorted in the context of illness. We know that one by-product of neurotic and psychotic indispositions, for instance, is a heightened self-consciousness of physical appearance or of its possible unpleasant effect on others. We know, too, that people seem to differ about the way in which they consider themselves protected or displayed by their bodies. Some feel walled in; some feel continually open to invasion. Such differences seem to be related to psychosomatic disturbances, but much remains to be discovered about these relationships.

Body, Mind, and Pain

The ground plan of the body makes for very definite opportunites and limitations within the domain of social relations. The fact that we have two eyes and a back, that we walk best upright and forward rather than sideways or backwards, that we have hands that can touch most of ourselves, though parts of it we can only see in a mirror, that a pattern of major orifices (quite apart from an invisible web of pores) facilitates a continuous exchange between ourselves and an environment which, among other things, includes other people—all provide the conditions within which social interaction must proceed, or on account of which it is undertaken.

Finally, the ground plan of the body provides us, if we so wish, with the paradoxical sense of both power and helplessness. Illness plays into both of these senses, sometimes with opposite effects. If for the moment we think of power as sheer physical strength or skill, bending to our will the physical world, then the self-conscious experience of being able, at will, to shake one's head or wiggle one's toes, to get up or lie down, can provide a sense of power and autonomy. The same actions, however, can be carried out without the action of our will: we can be hypnotized. The body, in other words, can be in our own control or that of others, and our knowledge of this fact helps to give us an experience of power. It also reminds us of the fact that in many ways we do not know how our decisions are translated into action. On the other hand, the body is equally subject to intrusion and influences over which we have no control. We can forestall certain of these through a familiar repertoire of preventive measures, but unless we seek them, attacks of appendicitis, or TB, or eczema, or the development of nearsightedness, happen to us, and they challenge our sense of autonomy. Interestingly enough, illness may itself lead to a cure that replaces a private sense of helplessness with a public sense of social domination; that is, we can

31

experience through illness a self-importance and self-consciousness that might have been closed to us under conditions of continuing health.

Finally, the act of fighting a physical condition or disability may afford us a sense of competence which, for all its derivations from our physical resources, comes to stand for the power of the self over the body. We would be inclined to argue that inherent in the experience of the body are at least the seeds of that troubling dichotomy of "body and mind," or mind and matter, which also persist, if often contradictorily, within the medical domain. Moreover, our separation of the ill from the well, for all its logical or scientific difficulties, has always been compounded by the further division between those ill in body from those ill in mind. The importance of these distinctions deserves special consideration, even if very brief.

ILLNESSES OF THE MIND

We can rail against the distinction between mind and body and regret the loss of the monistic, if magical, unity of the two that we attribute (probably wrongly) to some distant past; we can announce our new sophistication under various labels, including a concern with psychosomatic medicine, but the stubborn contrast between immediately felt thought (or awareness in general) and a dumb thereness of both the body and the external world remains. We must be content, for our purposes, to benefit from the tensions of this separateness.

In the West, emotional disturbances, especially when they assume dramatic and engrossing proportions, have traditionally forced themselves on the attention of society. The response of society to these disturbances has varied, and this variation, although orderly, has not fallen into a single line of progressive improvement of the treatment of the mentally ill, although in the short run this may seem to have been the case.

There has, however, been an extension of the activities of the medical profession, in line with its growing specialization. Illness has come to include the neuroses and psychoses, hysterias, epilepsies, and all the variations of retardation. This inclusiveness has been accompanied by a narrowing and a broadening of medical boundaries—both a dissociation of curing, as a professional enterprise, from the clinical activities of the clergy and other nonmedical helpers, and new modes of teamwork within medicine itself.

We no longer think of emotional disturbance as possession by demonic powers or by the devil, yet we witness a revived interest in counseling by the clergy, as well as by psychologists and others. Furthermore, with the specialization of psychiatry and neurology, emotional disturbances have become a special target for research and social reform as well as treatment, and as such they deserve special discussion in a separate book. In fact, social scientists interested in health have paid particular attention to mental hospitals, psychiatrists, and emotional disorders. Clearly, the explication of both human motives and social relations would seem to be assured if the self-conscious attention to personal histories and to the relation between therapists and patients—which are standard components of the cures of such disorders—can explicate them. In spite of the interests and practices that have emphasized the social and psychological aspects of emotional disturbances, there can be no denying their biological or somatic components, whatever their social cause. These illnesses, in the end, affect all aspects of our lives; they involve a perturbing impairment of our capacity to act as human beings: to work, to love, and to play. They interrupt our life in that created social world in which there must be, if it is to exist at all, some congruity between our images of ourselves and the images others have of us.

Much ink and exhortation have been used to des-

33

cribe man's inhumanity to man; madness and crime have presented favorite opportunities for the exercise of cruelty. Or so it seems in retrospect. Similarly, children and women, and in fact all weak minorities, be they ethnic, religious, racial, or social, have provided opportunities for some to vent their anger and for others to promote their brand of social reform. But what is cruelty? And, even more importantly for our purposes: what is madness? What is its relation to the domains of cure and of punishment? What is the bearing of these domains on madness?

Insane asylums, witch hunting, public provisions for the deranged, and the ambivalent support for those who would seek their reform have a long history that cannot be detailed here. This history, to oversimplify, has been suspended between several extremes: there are those who see illness in general, and a distraught mind in particular, as proofs of an immoral, or at least an imbalanced, life. It is not a long step from this position to the belief that the mad are in fact possessed by evil powers. The mad, in this view, do not constitute a medical, but rather a moral and religious problem.

Some have viewed the mad as possessed persons and thus to be feared; they have represented a dangerous connection with realms beyond the empirical world. Fear is close to enmity and hate, and so the mad, by this logic, became an enemy to be excluded, even to be killed. Among the early Greeks, in contrast, although not among the members of the Hippocratic circle, epilepsy was considered a sacred disease. Mental disturbance, after all, sustains a plausible connection to spiritual malaise. In the Mosaic tradition, mental disease, for all the acknowledgment of the fact that it was not a simple and unitary matter, remained a mystery. It was reprehensible or admirable, but it did not belong to the medical domain.

The Hippocratic tradition has sought to extend the medical domain and its concern with this world to include the management of depressions, epilepsies, and the deliria that sometimes accompany infections. In its effort to differentiate among madnesses, it has spoken of mania, melancholia, paranoia, and hysteria. Today we still use these terms, even if we use them differently and at times with essential misgivings. What to the Greeks was paranoia, to us would be a form of deterioration. Paranoia, that deep and negative tie to society, we would reserve for that extreme, persistent, and self-fulfilling attribution of enmity to others that becomes hardened into a destructive system. However, we do not know how much distrust is actually necessary, provided its proportions remain appropriately limited, for a sane life in society, but we have a sense for when it is too exaggerated. Indeed, many physical and mental illnesses might be conceived of as caricatures of body and mind, and hence also as caricatures of the arrangements through which we interact one with another.

Hysteria, to return to the Greeks, was actually not considered to be a mental disease in the strict sense. As it was only observed in women, a uterus, wandering about in the body, was considered to be its cause. Marriage was conceived as the most promising cure for hysteria, at least in the case of young girls. Thus, the sexual implications of this disorder have been recognized, if indirectly, for a very long time. The direct use of sexuality as an explanatory principle for emotional disturbances in general, and hysteria in particular, received its most masterful and controversial elaboration in the mind and writings of Freud. Preoccupation with hysteria in fact represented a crucial episode and minor revolution in the long tradition of concern with the modes of organization and disorder that characterize human personalities.

For our purposes it is enough to see in Freud's proposals a radical extension of Hippocrates' belief in the "natural" and "unsacred" character of disturbances of the mind. Freud's extension has both the merits and difficulties of beginning with a view of man as a biological entity, driven by natural yet opposing drives that are organized into a psychic economy called ego. That ego is deeply subject to its own imagination, even if it can also achieve self-knowledge and self-mastery through its use of reason. Reason binds it to an external world, but self-knowledge is also part of reason and part of the process of cure.

We have now arrived at a position that seems to be the opposite of the belief that the mentally ill are sacred or possessed, and as such "wholly other," possibly dangerous, and perhaps even to be killed. Our present naturalist-humanist position would have us think of physical and emotional, or normal and mad, as continuous conditions. It would, in opposition to unpalatable dichotomies, refer to these contrasts as matters of degree. What precisely this humanist belief means is not clear, except that it stresses the curability of mental disease, points to the self-fulfilling prophecy whereby we confirm, through imposed isolation in large mental hospitals, the emotional debilities partly engendered by earlier unplanned social isolation. A humanist belief robs emotional disturbances of their moral opprobrium, thus bringing them closer to clearly organic illnesses.

Within the professional domain, and outside, such a humanist view can again be divided into complementary, or rival, emphases. Some people, guided by an inclusive idea of nature, hope ultimately to find an organic explanation for all human illnesses, though not presumably for all human plights. Others, though acknowledging the biological character of human illnesses, would prefer to keep the front of inquiry wide. They would accordingly see human experiences as significant, dependent on the organism but never fully understandable in its terms. These people would then seek for the causes and consequences of the psychoses or neuroses in the domains of human motives, social arrangements, and cultural traditions. They would see these as providing different combinations of stress and support.

A given event, such as someone falling ill, always raises the possibility of choice: one can ignore it, or one can pay attention to it. One can choose to ask: How did it happen? or, What would happen if society never contained ill persons? As a member of society one may also ask: What can be done? and, What should be done? In any concrete circumstance such questions are much more elaborate, yet behind their complexities persists the simple fact that we live in a universe of distinctions. We do not live as though what surrounds us is an undifferentiated greyness of meaningless and insignificant happenings, happening to us. We may, for one reason or another, try to reach such a position, but our attempt would inevitably be nourished by the alternatives it seeks to escape.

To the extent to which we live in a world of meaning and distinction, the distinction between sane and mad, healthy and ill will accompany us. As we think about these, we will find them both elusive and continuous. We will perhaps only be really clear about the seriousness of the grosser forms of illness, and perhaps about sanity and health as necessary utopias, whereas between these extremes we will have doubts about what is sick and what is well. As we act, however, we will be forced to be more economical and to seek sharper distinctions. We will, as it were, close our ranks.

Broadly speaking, laymen seem to consider a wider range of behaviors normal than do most professionals, but once having withdrawn the word *normal* from their description of another's conduct, laymen are inclined to draw a distinction that implies discontinuity between well and ill. The radical difference between the normal and the mad, so conceived, helps buttress an unwillingness to assume much responsibility for such persons or to sustain much intimacy with them: let

37

the mad be cared for by those who can help them; let them be away from our company. Such an attitude seldom appears in pure form or in public, and it is most likely quite unequally spread through society. The more educated and the younger members of the laity seem more willing to entertain the idea that madness both reflects on the health of those around the affected person and constitutes a responsibility for more than a professional community. That community, in contrast with the laity, seeks sickness as a permanent possibility within anyone, and thus sees it more quickly, more ubiquitously.

The laity, of course, will not be at one in their views of madness. We should not be too surprised to find that in addition to the older and less educated, those who value personal excellence, effort, and self-control are less likely to be imbued with a sense of concern and responsibility for the mental illness of others than those who value service to the community.

To be in the presence of a mad person, someone not just temporarily beside himself, tired, nervous, or under stress, throws light upon the very anatomy of society. The deranged person represents unpredictability; he ceases to be understandable. One can find no simple explanation for the mad, be he psychotic or severely neurotic. One may demand of him that he "pull himself together," but he documents that he cannot do so. His symptoms, to use a necessary but misleading expression, seem stubborn, his demands insatiable; he constitutes an alternative interpretation of the world, and we, surrounding him, are unwilling to grant it.

Unpredictability makes social life more trying, and it is a personal threat because it reminds us of our own capacities for disturbance: the emotionally ill person's difference from us is an incomplete one. His unpredictability is an island in a sea of normalcy. His visions and attributions, his excessive activities or excessive withdrawals are in persistent ways

Body, Mind, and Pain

visible and external accomplishments of fantasies that remain half-acknowledged within ourselves.

We may abhor the thought that the mad should be locked into prisonlike hospitals, but we demand, nevertheless, that the community be protected from them. We declare that they should not be victims of custodial arrangements but beneficiaries of therapeutic communities; but at the same time we expect these communities to have walls, even if the openings in them are no longer to be locked.

One may be morally indignant about the treatment of the mentally ill, but that is to forget that many psychotics or otherwise emotionally disordered persons in our society are in fact kept within the protective, or destructive, web of a family or other constellation of people. In spite of this known holding power of society, however, one must acknowledge that there is in it a fairly strong disinclination to be or remain associated with the problem of mental illness. We expect the mad to be managed by the medical domain, yet we still think of them as sick in different fashion from the somatically ill. We may bridge this gap with a notion of "psychosomatic" ailments, but our images then form a triangle rather than a continuous straight line. There is a widespread tendency to "deny, isolate, and insulate mental illness,"[3] yet, at the same time, we are prepared to extend a psychological perspective to other modes of unacceptable or undesirable conduct such as delinquency and crime. At the same time, we seek to retain our commitments to notions of responsibility, and hence of punishment.

Today we look at those whom we call mad in several ways: as living criticisms of the damaging elements of society;

[3] See E. and J. Cumming, *Closed Ranks: An Experiment in Mental Health Education.* Cambridge: Harvard University Press, 1957, with special attention to Chapter VII, "A Patterned Response to a Form of Deviance and an Analysis of Its Function," pp. 112–134.

as necessary victims of certain stresses the absence of which might still exact a greater social and personal price; or as possible resources for which we have yet to find an adequate use. In a sense, the mad are both hostages to fortune and a challenge to our ingenuity.

Madness is often denied by the mad, who are frequently forced under protest to assume the role of being ill that others find apt for them. Because emotions and conceptions of the mad call into question what others wish to take as self-evident and appropriate, they are easily assimilated to the status of strangers. If we isolate the mad in hospitals, we may do so because we wish to make them familiar again; to leave them in the ordinary world—quite apart from the physical danger, which actually or putatively may be present—would be to act out a degree of tolerance for emotional conduct which our ideals of the self-controlled, reliable, striving, and rational man can hardly be expected to provide. To whose advantage it would be if our ideals and requirements were in fact different and allowed, say, for much more respect for visions and hallucinations is quite a different question.

The suffering that is intrinsic to emotional disturbance is not like a specific bodily pain; it is part of the very structure of the illness itself. Such illness, moreover, whatever its biological causes, enters deeply into one's relations to oneself and to others. It constitutes a reordering of these relations. Once begun, this reordering leads to further reordering in the face of the responses of those others on whom one depends, or who depend on one.

The modern view of emotional illness, however, tends to be assimilated to a medical tradition that has a successful history of struggling with somatic disturbance. Thus, neuroses and psychoses tend more often than not to be considered as medical entities rather than as different modes of engagement with others and oneself. This medical label further helps the sane to disengage themselves from the mad. On the other hand, our separation of the sane and the mad also gives the latter a holiday from the milieu in which they fell sick. When they have been at least partially restored in a milieu more nearly ordered to their requirements, they can, it is hoped, return as less vulnerable persons. Too often, of course, the intended cure further entrenches the disease.

Finally, the recognition of madness, like the recognition of crime, is part of the recognition of the openness of even the most closed society. It introduces a difference. It leads to one form of the contrast between heterodoxy and orthodoxy. Further, it provides a contrast between the ordinary and the extraordinary, the insider and the outsider, the mundane and the sacred. In the main, though, our penetration and cure of neuroses and psychoses have not reflected any sensitivity to their role in these social contrasts, but have taken the form of clinical and scientific exploration. Today we seem committed to reshaping the mad so that they can return to a predictable and engaged style of life rather than to the alternative, which is to extend the bounds of our social groupings to make greater room for those forms of madness that are neither sources of violence nor of demagoguery, and hence provide no permanent injury to social arrangements. Indeed, the potentiality of such mild madnesses gives life in society a permanently dramatic possibility.

PAIN

Pain takes many forms; it is part of more than illness.

. . . *in the records of all periods, misfortune has left more traces than happiness.* (Huizinga, *The Waning of the Middle Ages*)

It is surprising how few of the pains of men have entered their philosophies. (Simmel, *Fragmente und Aufsaetze*)

41

But we must limit ourselves to discussing, and that only in outline, the social patterning of the experience and expression of pain. This patterning includes, as well, the evaluation and imposition of pain.

Hannah Arendt reminds us in a book, aptly called *The Human Condition,* that the experience of "great bodily pain is at the same time the most private and least communicable of all."[4] We do not know whether this is empirically true, although we can reason cogently that pain, whatever its form or its intensity, seems indeed to adhere to the self. We may share our sorrow and so halve it, or share our joy and so double it, but we cannot share our pain. We cannot give our pain away, yet it may, when it is very intense, take us away from others, and from our environment. It may consume us entirely and thus incapacitate us for being in the world of things and of other persons.

The experience of pain, and of suffering, involves our images of the body and of ourselves, which, we assume, are constituted with the help of others and within society. Notions of pain and suffering, it should follow, will not be idiosyncratic, but will exhibit some orderly variation within and between societies. Ideas about pain should be affected by the great cleavages that run through social arrangements: age, ethnicity, sex, and education. Concepts of pain should also involve some of the fundamental assumptions concerning that which is desirable and that which is inevitable by which people come to order the direction of their experience and the goals of their lives.

Certainly pain is more than a specific bodily sensation that can be fully accounted for by some external event. We see in pain a mode of experiencing or anticipating what we expect to affect us. The source and place of our pain may

[4] H. Arendt, *The Human Condition.* Garden City, New York: Doubleday, 1959, p. 46.

have no simple physical connection; neither does pain need to be, no matter how specifically we can point to its bodily source, entirely a reaction to a definite bodily injury. It can be a somatic reaction to an injury to our essential selves: deep or acute grief, as we know, is more specific than a hurtful sadness, and we can feel grief in a specific site—the pit of our stomach.

We can feel our aches and pains with more or less attention, knowing them to "be" in specific parts of our bodies or to concern our embodied selves. We can describe them more or less aptly or misleadingly. We tend to see them as signs of our illness, except when they are the illness itself, as in an emotional disturbance whose pains of anxiety constitute the illness we wish to lose. Pain as such we distinguish by form and severity. When pain becomes crystallized into either temporary or chronic elements of our experience, it also becomes subject to a variety of social evaluations. It becomes the occasion for a special pattern of social conduct—consolation and compassion.

In general, in our society, we bring toward pain an optimistic and an activist bias. We do not expect people to seek pain; rather, we expect to be increasingly able to escape it. Among other things, medicine is our institutionalized insurance toward that end. Yet pain, in its specific and somatic manifestations, is not a totally separate phenomenon; it is continuous with a long line of other misfortunes, and it is part of our apprehension of actual and potential injury, of too much or too little. Once pain occurs, it raises at least these three questions: What does it mean? How can or should I express this experience in the company of others? Why does it happen, and why to me?

In spite of our general disposition to avoid pain, it can be sought as punishment, that is deliberately imposed rather than deliberately reduced. Further, even when we seek treatment rather than accepting pain as punishment, it can be

43

increased as a by-product of cure. The sites in which pain occurs, moreover, are greeted with variable compassion, and thus variably viewed by others as punishment or plight. In our society, for instance, pain arising from the genitalia or the rectum tends to be more hedged about and thus less subject to the exchange of sympathy than burns and fractures, or pains in the abdomen or chest.

Within this scheme of things, Mark Zborowski's findings on four groups of patients in a Veterans hospital provide the beginnings of some further understanding.[5] The patients were of Jewish, Italian, Irish, and "Old American" origins. In the main they suffered from herniated discs and spinal lesions. The Jewish and Italian patients, in the eyes of their doctors, exaggerated their pain. Such a medical assumption raises many issues. It suggests that given types of somatic disturbances cause given amounts of pain and that therefore the claims of one patient can validly be compared with those of others. This assumption suggests that there are norms that govern how much pain it is appropriate to feel, or at least to express, in response to this or that injury. Such norms seem to deny the subjectivity of pain. At least they raise the question: How genuine are the patient's claims of pain? The expression of pain, in other words, has social consequences and is therefore socially regulated. The experience of pain, on the other hand, though engendered in the sense meant here only within social beings, is inward and private and reminds us that we are bounded creatures whose boundaries can be invaded or destroyed. By contrast, then, Jewish and Italian patients seemed to make much more of their pain than the Irish and Old Americans; they let its existence be well known. More-

[5] M. Zborowski, "Cultural Components in Responses to Pain," *Journal of Social Issues,* 1952, *8*(4). The whole study of which this is a part is now available in Zborowski, *People in Pain.* San Francisco: Jossey-Bass, 1969.

over, these patients conceived of their pain differently from the Irish and Old American patients.

There were other differences. The Italians isolated their pain and wanted it removed. Once out of pain, they were satisfied, and their concern dried up. The Jewish patients, in contrast, saw their pain as a sign of a more generally disturbed state of affairs, and their concern about it went deeper and involved not only their present condition but also their future state. Indeed, in referring to strong pain, Jewish patients used the word *yessurim*, "worry," which revealed their anxiety. The experience of pain, furthermore, brought out different attitudes towards doctors. Italian patients typically had confidence in medical care, especially when their doctors were successful in relieving them of pain. Jewish patients saw no reason for suspending their doubts about their health even in the face of medical success, unless their doctors could help dissolve their underlying anxieties about their biological states.

Old Americans, in contrast with Italians and Jews, were also concerned with pain, but solely in order to report about it. It was as if these patients viewed their bodies at a distance in order that their objectivity could help their doctors to restore them to health. To groan and to moan seemed pointless to them, for it would, after all, "not help anybody." Pain is to be borne, until it is removed or reduced. But what of unbearable pain? For the Old Americans its rigors were to be suffered in private if not in silence, and therefore great pain meant withdrawal from society. Old American patients, like the Jewish ones, experienced the anxiety of pain, but they balanced their concern with it by a faith in the accomplishments and efficacy of the whole medical domain, including hospitals.

Such stoical behavior can be simulated by people whose attitudes are privately more pessimistic than appears on the outside. Patients who are the descendents of immigrants,

Health and Healing

for example, may engage in behavior like that described for Old Americans while concealing some of the attitudes just described for Italian patients. Furthermore, occupation and education complicate the patterns of ethnicity. Headaches, for example, plague intellectuals more frequently than manual workers, as we might expect. With herniated discs, the situation is reversed.

On the whole, the more educated are also more health-conscious than the less educated, yet the less-educated Old American or Jewish patient is more health-conscious than the more-educated Italian patient. More-educated patients, however, tend to feel more restricted in the spontaneous expression of their sense of pain and discomfort. Self-control and the self-consciousness that education brings seem to go together, at least as ideals.

The expression of pain is not an isolated process; it provides opportunities for the exercise of passive resignation or of active mastery; as such, it engages the ideals of both masculinity and femininity. Pain is more than the absence of pleasure: it represents the experience of injury, and therefore, when collected into a pattern of suffering, pains may even represent a sense of something being positively right as well as wrong. There are potent cultural traditions in Western society that would have us not only balance pleasure and pain and pay with the latter for the former, but would also have us feel that we have done our best only "when it hurts." To be sure, there are other, perhaps equally potent, traditions that would reject such a view outright, label it neurotic, and give us the right to pursue, if not happiness, then certainly fun. Some modicum of resignation, however, is provided for in most social arrangements, for most of them contain, and perhaps even engender, more pain and injury than can be balanced with pleasure, or be reduced by fun.

Given this ambivalence to pain, medicine, including

46

psychiatry, attempts to gain or maintain an order of well-being, as distinct from a state of grace, salvation, or happiness that confines pain and suffering to the realms of the body's functioning on the one hand and the self's decisions and awareness on the other. To accomplish this, medicine seeks to keep separate notions of pain and guilt, evil and injury, tribulation and injustice, insult and sin even though these pairs are easily associated.

Ultimately, the invasion of the self by pain provides an opportunity for the experience of both deprivation and restoration. It provides the opportunity of surviving a crisis. On some occasions this can mean a second birth, or, at least, access to rare insights such as accompany death and birth. In Western society, the medical domain, perhaps in reaction to religious institutions, makes professional aid available at death and birth. Neither event can be left unattended; both are crises for more than those being born or dying.

Pregnancy, whether accompanied by malaise or not, is generally associated with a medical regime. For some elements of the population, it is thus likely to have features in common with illness. The end of pregnancy is at least potentially a crisis to be attended by professionally schooled persons. The pains of labor and of birth, moreover, help to differentiate women from men and, perhaps more poignantly, child-bearing women from other women. In North America, for the most part, we expect births to take place within hospitals. Arrangements for this are quite varied, yet they include the chance of mothers in labor struggling in the presence of other struggling mothers whom they have never seen before and whom they may never see again. In pain, as in few things, the private and the public realm can meet.

Death, which is the end of pain, yields both the pain of dying and the sorrow of surviving, yet we know we must honor the dead, or else life would become cheap. We must arrange for both their disposal and their replacement. These sorrows we expect; their absence would itself cause us concern. Their presence, felt as grief and expressed through the cultural forms of mourning, thrives on a compound of sentiments. That compound includes, so clinicians and others tell us, anger at the loss, fear lest one may have contributed to it, fear that the dead may indeed survive and haunt us, pleas for support in our loss, irritation that drives such support away, and anger at oneself because a relation to another has been disrupted while one's sentiments toward him still thrive.

Our society makes some room for the resolution of these sentiments by allowing the aggrieved to withdraw, at least temporarily, from ordinary obligations. Such a withdrawal allows for the expected expressions of grief. As with illness, withdrawal through grief is a suspension of some of one's social obligations so that one may be free, perhaps with the help of others, to concentrate on personal and emotional matters. Such concentration is, in part at least, the discharge of an obligation. Grief is work. Like work, it can be well or badly done, either eventually dissipating or, alternatively, spreading the disruption begun by the loss.

Death, certain as fact but uncertain in its arrival, is at once the end of our pains and a source of them. Yet the certainty of death is not for all of us equivalent to the finality of death. We ask doctors, coroners, and some others to pronounce us dead, but not to pronounce on the character of death. That character has been quite variously imagined, but it is not known what specific difference knowledge of it may make to the process of dying; we do not know whether a person sees death as a passage from one world to another or as the very end of all. Dying, whatever its accompanying complications, fears, or serenities may be, does not offer just one or the other of these two alternatives. The other world may, after all, be considered in benign or in other terms:

Very few cultures picture the next world as a better one or as one in which the divine balance of justice is redressed. In many cases reunion is either not envisaged or is not presented in attractive terms. Even the threat of punishment after death is comparatively seldom used as a sanction to produce moral behavior on this earth. Finally, one can hardly consider immortality, in the strict sense, as a pan-human concept. Almost all peoples have conceived of some continuation, of something that was not extinguished with the last beat of the heart. But this is not invariably felt to be permanent. A gradual extinction is often portrayed, or a sudden annihilation after so many generations or other fixed period. When the soul is thought to be imperishable, personal immortality does not necessarily follow. The soul-stuff may be merged with that of others or in natural forces.[6]

Collectively, the curative domain stands at the rim of death—announcing it, helping with the traditions of disposal, perhaps easing the agonies of dying. Interestingly enough, today we do not publish books on the craft of dying, though we publish on the art of managing most other passages, from birth and love to retirement and old age.

Death is linked to pain only some of the time. We may die of old age, peacefully in our sleep, feeling fulfilled. More of us will think of death as an interruption, as a symbol of our permanent insufficiency. Yet, for all our dread of it, death may interrupt our pains, even the pain of growing old. In this way, the fact of death gives a general character to all our pleasures and pains. It endows them with limits, and points up the degree to which health is concerned with the integrity of boundaries.

[6] C. Kluckhohn, *Culture and Behavior*. Glencoe, Ill.: Free Press, 1962, p. 137.

3

The Medical
Domain

M edicine is both a tradition and a profession. On
the one hand, its tradition involves an application and extension of specialized knowledge that is applied to unique individual cases. Medicine is to use knowledge for helping others.
It must prevent illness, it must relieve pain, it must restore
health, and, in modern society, it must guide the transition

50

from the womb to the world or from the world to the grave. Medicine is a profession allied to the skepticism and experimental neutrality of science. The growth of science has been to the advantage of medicine, and the growth of medicine can no longer systematically proceed apart from the growth of science.

On the other hand, medicine must take effect in the practical world. It must be practiced on people. It cannot proceed as if the body were only a machine, although its procedures depend on knowledge that derives from the use of such a perspective. Emotional disturbances aside, medicine clearly intervenes in a natural order, but this natural order has itself been endowed with meaning by patients and sufferers. For example, the medical profession has accepted the meaning its own patients bestow upon nature, calling for the reduction of pain and the enhancement of well-being. Apart from chronic illness, medicine also intervenes in situations of crisis. It must provide steady help when those whom it helps are unsteady. Its steadiness, as we have seen, depends in large part upon specialized knowledge and on the maintenance of considerable social distance between physician and patient. At the same time, its help often depends on a doctor's capacity for compassion. In short, the medical tradition, as a professional one, is concerned with doing its best for the sake of others, but at the same time it typically depends on income derived from those others, quite independent of its success. The contrast and potential contradiction between welfare and profit is not a simple one. Doctors have more than one patient, at the same time that they are masters of scarce resources; they therefore face the problem of just distribution, and they cannot be exclusively guided by a simple economic formula based on the patient's ability to pay.

Even if each doctor succeeds in allocating his time and resources fairly, a solution for the best allocation of the total

51

medical resources of a society to its medical needs is clearly not automatically available. Such a distribution calls for wider perspectives which cannot issue from the medical tradition, with its dependence on an institutional autonomy within which doctors and patients can choose each other.[1] Still, the variety of social and economic distributive arrangements compatible with such freedom is greater than the defenders of special arrangements for medical practice will sometimes admit.

The medical domain as a whole balances reliance on clinical experience with reliance on basic research. The former is organized around personal knowledge and taught by teachers to pupils; the latter, though issuing from the same realm, is organized around experiment and statistics through which a precise knowledge concerning the definite beginnings of our ignorance is sought. From this contrast, a further contrast emerges: the expectation that physicians be both specialists who stand in a technical tradition and at the same time be cultivated and learned men and women. If they successfully embody these two traditions, they are not likely to consider as alien anything that is human, and their interest in illness would be given form by their knowledge of the rich alternatives for the uses of health.

Illness, like pain, is experienced by those who undergo it as adhering to the self, and although it can be shared and discussed, it cannot be given away. Those, like doctors, who come to participate in others' plights come to participate in others' affairs. This participation yields a process of mutual appropriation of skills between doctors and other helpers who attend on people's plights. Such an exchange of skill leads to various patterns of exclusion, in which certain medical activi-

[1] With the reservations which we will put forth in the forthcoming section. (Editor's note: It is not quite clear what was intended by this note.)

ties, such as performing surgery or certifying deaths, belong only to doctors and cannot be taken from them or given away.

Taken in the round, the domain of medicine is a product of various traditions; its contrasting origins still linger to enrich its practices.

This book is written in and about an urban and industrial society. We call such a society modern and experience it as complex. A complex society is *differentiated,* and this abstract word refers to a number of related concrete facts, chief among them being division of labor. This division has two levels; it involves the separation of the domain of remunerated work from the domain of home, family, and relatives, because industrial, as distinct from agricultural or nomadic, economies create a journey to work; and second, it involves complicated occupational systems. The complication of the occupational sphere involves the proliferation of many varieties of work. Associated with both the separation of the occupational world from the sphere of family life and the differentiation of the occupational world, are the partial segregation of the major domains of society itself and the increasing dependence of society on technology. These and other facts converge to subject an increasing number of social arrangements to a continuous and often accelerating pattern of social changes.

Contrasting present and past, it would be false either to see a distant and apparently simple past as a paradise of small human groupings enjoying genuine and unified consensus, or to compound the error by seeing a simpler past as a brutish and fearful world deprived of the knowledge, comforts, and securities of the present day. Similarly, it would be false not to recognize the huge complexity and vast accomplishments of knowledge and know-how that constitute our society.

As part of the proliferation of recognizably different

53

social domains, modern society includes the conspicuous establishment of a far-flung domain of health. This domain encom-
passes the prevention and cure of illness, as well as complicated
economic arrangements for the provision of medical care for
increasingly large and heterogeneous populations. The internal
differentiation of the medical domain involves two sets of contrasts: first, the art of clinical practice contrasted with the
pursuit of experimental and laboratory investigation; and
second, the two-person clinical encounter contrasted with the
large institution such as the pharmaceutical industry, medical
technology (as represented by operating procedures), and the
huge bureaucracies that sometimes administer medical care.

The establishment of such a complex medical domain
involves the partial dissociation of matters of illness from still
other domains such as religious institutions, and all practices
concerned with the salvation of men's souls. The detailed facts
of this dissociation are rich and complicated and are part of
that overall shift in attitudes and arrangements that constitutes
modernization.

In the main, we must take these matters for granted;
here we simply wish to stress that:

First, the autonomy of the medical domain, like the
autonomy of the legal domain, proceeds within a broad context of moral neutrality. Doctors and nurses treat the ill without regard to religious, political, or other commitments. They
treat them within a tradition that derives its substance from
the elaboration of clinical experience and the application of
science to human plight.

Second, such moral neutrality is in many respects incomplete. Hospitals are frequently integrated with one or
another of the main religious traditions of Western society,
although their admission policies do not usually impose religious tests. Aspects other than the conditions of the patient's
illness, such as occupational or military status, do, however,

54

explicitly affect his chances of medical care. Nor is moral neutrality to be misunderstood as an actual claim of equal accessibility of medical resources to the sick of a society in complete disregard of their ability to pay, their social status, their ethnicity, or their place of residence.[2] Moral neutrality is concerned with the individual patient and refers to a governing tendency, once a professional or clinical encounter has been arranged, to pursue this encounter as though illness and suffering were phenomena to be understood rather than specifically judged and punished. Moral neutrality demands the conquest of individual illnesses, once care is undertaken, to the best of available professional abilities.

Third, the autonomy of the medical domain is, paradoxically, contingent on qualities within those other spheres of society, religion, education, occupation, and kinship from which it has been partially separated. Autonomy, in other words, does not mean utter independence. Rather, it means a deliberate segregation of medically restitutive or preventive measures from other forms of human influence and aid.

Fourth, such segregation exists alongside a cross-cutting tendency in which elements of clinical practice are also found, though differently organized, in other human encounters such as religious conversions, successful pilgrimages to religious shrines, and the resolution through human interaction of inner plights imposed by and in childhood. However, the major organization of the medical domain sets it off from institutions with similar or resonant elements.

Modern society, as civil society, binds us into nations, and the medical and nursing professions reflect this fact. Most of the materials of this book apply in the first instance to North American conditions, although the study of illness and

[2] A community study by A. B. Hollingshead and F. C. Redlich, *Social Class and Mental Illness*. New York: Wiley, 1958, investigates the unequal accessibility to psychiatric services.

Health and Healing

cure requires not only comparison among nations but also the recognition of an international scientific and professional community. Illness, after all, though unequally distributed in time and place and often meaningfully aligned with social cleavages such as class, occupation, sex, and age, knows at the same time no simple historic, social, and national barriers. Medical knowledge, in other words, being constituted by the discoveries of science, contains a strain toward universality. Yet we know that the arrangements of medical care are often jealously guarded as matters of "local rights." A proper view of the medical domain must therefore always be bifocal. It must concern itself both with the self-contained and professional character of medical practice and with the association of this practice with the other domains of society.

Manifestly, the medical domain does not develop in a single and simple line of growing knowledge and competence, even though larger numbers of people, certainly within the Western world, are considerably better off, physically speaking, than was true in, say, the tenth century A.D. If the image of a straight line will not serve the facts, the image of a spiral might. Knowledge concerning illness has undoubtedly been dramatically expanded. This expansion has involved the depersonalization of illness because it has called for an alliance between the clinic and the laboratory, between many bedsides and numerous research institutes. The alliance is fruitful, yet not easy. It is part of a long process that involves the continuous complication and refinement of medical practice.

To a very large extent, illness has become a matter of professional rather than lay management. Variations of such management in the form of Christian Science, on the one hand, and of folk medicine, on the other, are, after all, another side of the professionalization of cure. This professionalization, which also includes specialization, is always associated with illness, even when the latter is considered primarily as a moral

56

phenomenon rather than as an impersonal and natural occurrence.

Fifth, the process of depersonalizing illness revealed it as a natural phenomenon, subject to laws of cause and effect and requiring the understanding of the nature of organisms and of the relations among organisms. This view has produced an advance of knowledge and understanding, especially during the last fifty years. Recently, however, we have tended to return to the pre-nineteenth-century notions that stressed the importance of human experience and conduct. In an earlier day, these notions helped to give impetus to magical practice, but the contemporary emphasis on psychosomatic medicine with its interest in emotional disturbance has reintroduced into the medical domain what has never been absent but has often been kept hidden. This raw emphasis is a concern with individual motives, social relations, and institutional arrangements, as these influence the well-being of individual personalities housed in bodies.

Sixth, our knowledge and understanding of health and illness as characteristic states of individuals have been enlarged or revised through the tension and vitality provided by a continuous controversy. Some of the elements of this controversy are:

Illness is a phenomenon to be mastered through knowledge or practice, but illness is also an aspect of the limitation of life. Together with aging and death, illness must be accepted in quite a number of its manifestations.

Fluctuations of well- and ill-being are primarily individual matters, but individual states are always affected by the states of other individuals as well as by those social arrangements that make us mutually dependent members of society.

Illness in all of its manifestations (including mental disorder) is a natural phenomenon to be understood through the combined resources of the natural and biological sciences, but no human phenomena, even when they involve the working of a natural order, can fully be known or understood in terms of the tradition of the natural and biological sciences. Rather, they require the growth of the so-called social sciences and of the humanities.

The curing of illness is an art involving primarily bedside and clinical teaching, an art that is nourished on the knowledge of basic sciences, though it requires skill and acumen that cannot be replaced by laboratory experiments. Still, medical research, as a systematic rather than clinical endeavor concerned with limited and isolatable phenomena, is an indispensable resource of the medical domain.

Medicine seeks to combine a rational tradition with an empirical and clinical one. The first would observe particular manifestations of illness in specific individuals, but the latter seeks general principles that could apply to particular cases.

The tradition and substance of medical thought include various images of the "ultimate" character of the human body. Through a variety of preferences for explanations cast in terms of fluid humors or solid cells, various concepts of harmony and conflict, and a proliferation of analogies between bodies and machines, the single craft of curing has led to quite various conceptions of nature, person, and society. The medical domain, therefore, like the sphere of religion, has come to have both its sects and its established doctrines. In a complex, differentiated society, it is a complex, differentiated domain.

SPECIALIZATION

A profession, like a society, becomes more complicated if it bases its existence in knowledge and technology because it is then bound to undergo accelerating social change. We should therefore expect the healing professions to be faced with repeated compromises, each in itself productive of further issues to be resolved. This succession of compromises is driven on by two contrasting demands: the demand for enough monolithic unity of the profession to provide medicine with an identity, common traditions, and a sense of excellence, and the simultaneous demand for a technical specialization meant to provide a single profession with a division of labor that can, in turn, implement the general purposes of the whole.

The structure and history of the Roman Catholic Church and that of the medical profession provide certain parallels. The priest has a choice: while subscribing to one creed, he can either be a member of an order primarily involved in a variety of administrative or teaching positions, or he can choose the complex pattern of parish work. The medical profession offers to its entrants a similar choice, although at the moment it is more a series of national enterprises than a single world community with "one creed." It is identified, however, with a general body of knowledge and competence while sustaining a rich complexity of specialties which, in turn, have quite different relations to this general medical tradition. Specialization, of course, is not a recent phenomenon. When shamans heal the sick, they are not considered interchangeable one with another: their command over the spirit world is unequal and different. It is the acceleration and prominence of specialization that are modern.

In the realm of health, modern specialization is sustained by a combination of situations:

In a measure it is an outgrowth of "localism," that is, the recognition and experience of the body as a configuration of parts. The ears, nose, and throat, the internal organs, the extremities, the heart, and the brain have all become subject to specialized bodies of knowledge. Such knowledge, in turn, yields its complementary traditions of skill.

A cross-cutting form of specialization in the form of surgery, internal medicine, public health, dermatology, orthodontics, and many others also generates traditions, groupings, and self-conceptions that tend to expand specialization into vested interests. Often these are made visible through special professional associations and journals. Nurses and doctors thus generally think of themselves less in generic terms, as nurses and doctors, and more in particular terms, as public health nurses, surgeons, obstetricians, and the like. In one sense, even the general practitioner is a breed apart, a family doctor.

With the growth of knowledge comes an advance in notions of excellence. We come to expect more. Regarding health, pain, and illness in the West today, we almost take it for granted that we shall not die in infancy, that medical care will be available to us in the form of doctors, nurses, laboratories, and hospitals, and that our wives will survive the birth of our progeny. Standards of excellence are, however, not a simple reflection of our capacities. We often expect, if not perfection, more than is yet possible. Our clinical encounters may, therefore, demand a lessening of our hopes, as well as a battle with inappropriate resignation. Yet even when less can be done for us than we had hoped or had been led to expect, the healing professions collectively possess resources that no single member can make his own in one lifetime. Specialization is a response to this fact. It sustains mastery by narrowing what is to be grasped. Only through specialization can standards of excellence prevail. Dilettantism is the extreme alternative to specialization, which, in short, constitutes a mode of mastery over a tradition that as a whole can no longer be mastered and that, by its nature and the demands put upon it, is subject to accelerating change.

Specialization that divides the body into parts and the profession into sections yields both high levels of care and new obstacles. The latter arise from the essential unity and coherence of individuals and of social arrangements. When medical care yields the increasing division of labor that grows out of specialization, it requires new patterns through which the divided laborers can also work in concert. This requirement leads to two divergent developments: first, the grouping of specialists in various kinds of clinics along with the establishment of complex, and often large, institutions that draw on the services of a wide range of specialists and the development of various kinds of regional and community health facilities; and, second, a reemphasis of the role of the general practitioner as a family doctor coordinating, for the benefit of patients, the technical and specialized services of the medical domain. This latter development both balances the centrifugal tendencies of specialization and at the same time yields new specialties, especially in matters of administration. Thus, as healing becomes technically specialized, it also becomes subject to the services of further specialists, including administrators. In this way, healing comes to be composed of several dimensions at once: technical procedures, human involvement with clients (of whom the patient is only one), and social relations with others, including colleagues, who together constitute the healing domain to which the sick seek temporary access, or from which they are to be released.

The patterns of medical specialization, and their association with large medical centers, teaching hospitals, and universities, clearly depend on a complex urban (or even metropolitan) culture. Such a culture includes a degree of population mobility and heterogeneity which militates against the older pattern of "family doctors."

The specialization of the wider society further adds to the principles of specialization within the domain of healing. The marriage of medical care with military, industrial, and educational institutions illustrates this further cross-cutting of specialization.

The requirements of professional identity affect the extent of specialization. In a contemporary medical class about

61

Health and Healing

to graduate from medical school, about seventy-five out of every one hundred students questioned were planning a career involving specialty practice. Ten per cent or so expected to teach or to do research. The rest looked forward to general practice.[3] The decision for specialization, moreover, grows within the medical school itself. At the beginning of their medical school careers, students are not in a position to make specific commitments concerning later plans, and so they keep themselves open and flexible. As they learn more medicine, they also recognize more clearly the complexity of medical practice and their own abilities to cope with some complexities and not with others. Specialization, once recognized as a legitimate pattern, helps to match individual capacities and professional possibilities. This matching is, of course, not only a question of a student's preferences and of knowledge; to some extent it also involves his actual performance in medical school, which leads his teachers, subtly or otherwise, to influence him away from or toward specialization.

The process of specialization creates countervailing efforts. In medicine these include the attempt to strengthen the role of the general practitioner. Ironically, the growth of one medical specialty, psychiatry, is one cause of this attempt. Increasingly we accept the presumption that emotional indispositions are a component of most forms of illness. Such a view strengthens the wish to see the "case" as a whole person without, however, becoming personally involved with him. Talk about the patient as "a whole person" can be pious and hackneyed, but it nevertheless expresses a bewildered displeasure at the segregation of patients into the spheres of the

[3] P. L. Kendall and H. C. Selvin, "Tendencies Toward Specialization in Medical Training," in R. K. Merton, G. G. Reader, and P. L. Kendall (Eds.), *The Student Physician.* Cambridge, Harvard University Press, 1957, pp. 153–174. See especially Table 14 and footnote on p. 156.

specialist's competence, while hiding the fact that we wish to continue to enjoy all the advantages that only specialization can provide.

Many issues lie buried here. We know that each patient moves in and out of his illness with the help or hindrance of patterns of response that were constituted in the past. Yet we are still debating, and shall continue to debate, how the past can or cannot be superseded by the present, and to what extent general modes of experiencing rather than specific events become the principles out of which our present responses are constructed. We can be sure, too, that organizations in which we must work and the circles in which we play will help to yield both our plight and our recovery.

The historic course of increasing specialization within the domain of healing is by no means a straight line interrupted only by attempts at maintaining the dignity and importance of the general practitioner. Modern medicine, for instance, has had to overcome a long-standing division between physicians and surgeons, in which the latter lacked professional respectability. Both are now within the professional community, and surgery, moreover, commands preeminent respect, at least in the eyes of the public. Not only does the standing of the various specialties shift within the profession, but the laity also distributes its attention and prestige unequally, and in a different way from the profession itself. In the meantime, new specialties such as space medicine emerge, sometimes almost unnoticed.

In general, specialists tend to be economically better off than general practitioners. One must distinguish, however, between general practice as a life career and general practice as a chapter in a doctor's biography, to be followed by specialization.

Specialization is here to stay, and will grow; but increasingly it will be accompanied by various devices intended to coordinate the services of specialists for the sake of the patient. Diverse social and medical services as well as new methods of collating information about patients' medical histories are some of the resources for maintaining "continuity of care" within a division of labor evolved for the provision of care.

MEDICAL EDUCATION

Professions are monopolies. They seek to restrict activities in which they profess competence to those who are duly licensed to perform them. Litigation, curing, nursing, engineering, teaching, and other such undertakings can only be formally carried on by those who have been permitted to do so by others who are already members in good standing of their profession. Professions must not only induct newcomers and make them welcome, but they must also face problems of aging, death, and expansion.

In principle, professions could let newcomers come from any quarter, merely asking of them that they pass one or more examinations designed to establish their competence. Yet, especially in the cases of medicine, law, and nursing, professional practice requires more than easily measurable or examinable technical knowledge: it demands clinical experience not only to learn the less palpable "art" of medicine, but also to become a conforming member of the society of doctors. Under present conditions, professional practice requires expensive formal education; medicine, nursing, and medical research, as full-time careers, thus require the maintenance of such institutional arrangements as faculties of medicine and schools of nursing, which provide some members of the profession with a career of teaching or research.

The contemporary pattern of the education of doctors and nurses is a mixture of old and new arrangements. The pattern is, moreover, in a permanent state of change. Medical education has become a university enterprise, yet not wholly so. It includes both preclinical and clinical training and, as a rule, a fairly standardized curriculum, ranging from the "basic sciences," biochemistry, bacteriology, physiology, and anatomy, to clinical specialties such as internal medicine, surgery, and psychiatry. Such a curriculum clearly demands the use of such clinical facilities as hospitals, out-patient departments, mental hospitals, and laboratories. Although these facilities must serve more than a university public, they make of medical education a distinct professional enterprise in which the student engages "as a whole" as he is prepared for a career. Few study medicine for the sake of a general education. In contrast, some study law, not to practice it, but to prepare themselves for a future in business or politics. Similarly, nursing is sometimes less than a lifetime commitment; for a few it is merely an adjunct to marriage and motherhood.

The standardization of the medical and nursing curricula requires agreement on a sequence of substantive fields and on the relative amount of time formally to be devoted to each. The curricula, moreover, with their complicated schedules, timetables, "block systems," and other formal arrangements, demand bureaucratic expertise. These are obvious facts, yet they constitute part of the complicated process necessary for transforming a layman into a member of a profession who can help others after him to be likewise transformed. The setting of this process varies among institutions. Although there are acknowledged differences among medical schools, their precise nature is not easy to assess and is obscured by irrelevant comparisons. (Individuals, of course, may transcend the limitations of their training or may fail to absorb the full benefits of it and hence not be representative.) Yet, if medical schools and schools of nursing differ, they differ only within limits, for professional medical education is carried on with the help of resources that are themselves accredited by nationally representative bodies.

As an enterprise, professional education[4] is devoted to the creation of future doctors or nurses whose conditions of practice will in some respects be quite different from those familiar to their teachers. Professional education also prepares people for more than one kind of career. Medical education, as we have noted, seeks to teach both systematic scientific information and clinical skills within definite limits of time, but the range of information deemed necessary for a properly trained medical student is itself growing. Medicine is, after all, as Robert K. Merton reminds us, "at heart a polygamist becoming wedded to as many of the sciences and practical arts as prove their worth."[5] The mates are multiplying, even if the older and earlier among them protest against such new arrivals as psychology and sociology.

Under these circumstances, it is no accident that medical education is now firmly established in universities, where a wealth of clinical information and experience can be transformed into a more economic form through inquiry, in contrast to an older and more casual empiricism. Indeed, medical education is being forced to be more systematic, and thus

[4] There is a growing body of knowledge on professional education and socialization. For perspectives on medical socialization, see, for instance, H. S. Becker and J. W. Carper, "The Development of Identification with an Occupation," *American Journal of Sociology,* 1956, *61*(4), pp. 289–298; H. S. Becker and B. Geer, "Student Culture in Medical School," *Harvard Educational Review,* 1958, *28*(1), pp. 70–80; E. C. Hughes, "The Making of a Physician," *Human Organization,* 1955, *14* (4), pp. 21–25; R. K. Merton, G. G. Reader, and P. L. Kendall (Eds.), *The Student Physician.* Cambridge: Harvard University Press, 1957.

[5] R. K. Merton, "Some Preliminaries to a Sociology of Medical Education," in Merton, et al., p. 32.

"scientific," in order to do justice to its own accomplishments, which have accumulated at such high speed during the last three hundred years. The very extension of the scientific basis of modern medical practice points up the fact that the ill who seek help and the well who seek the maintenance of their health maintain their somatic assets and liabilities within the supporting, or damaging, surroundings of both a personal world and an environment of social arrangements.

Medical education today, therefore, faces these questions: How can the advances of medical knowledge be incorporated into an already demanding and crowded curriculum? How can the "same" curriculum at once provide systematic knowledge concerning the pathology of the human organism, and clinical experience with the management of actually ill persons, as well as clinically relevant perspectives on the character of individuals and institutions?

As one examines studies of professional education, a number of impressions emerge. Schools of medicine and nursing are worlds unto themselves; they are, in the words of one medical student, "closed societies with 'ideals and gods' of their own." Such schools include only those who wish to prepare themselves for full-time participation in the medical domain. Schools of nursing, when they involve residential living, are even more inclusive than medical schools, guarding the private lives of their charges and keeping them close to their places of work. Within this closed society, established members of a profession help others to cease being laymen. Withdrawing from the laity perhaps involves, as Everett Hughes suggests, a separation amounting to alienation.

The process of professionalization requires a deliberate division of labor among teachers, students, patients, and later, nurses, residents, and others. All these share common standards, but they also develop various "subcultures." Each subgroup develops a working consensus that helps to define the problems to be faced and to select the solutions to be preferred. These subcultures, among other functions, provide rules for cooperation and competition, help define what to study and what to neglect, and form the students into a social unit in the sense of generating a solidarity that marks off one graduating class from another.

Students, of course, are guided by both previous attitudes and present advice; they face fairly definite and objective demands. Students also face contrary admonitions arising in personal differences among their faculty. Ultimately, they must decide on the qualities of a "good" physician or a "good" nurse. These qualities involve a series of balances between conflicting demands.

Professional education, especially in medicine, includes the experience of being overwhelmed. It is education in professional mastery of a large and growing field, which, in fact, cannot any longer be mastered. This sense of being overwhelmed is encouraged by the persistent division of medical education into a preclinical and a clinical phase. Although this pattern is from time to time experimentally varied, it is the essential and underlying one, and as such it exposes students to highly developed knowledge about localized pathology, to dissection and other forms of reduction of the organism into its component parts; in thus exposing them, it strengthens the view that specialization is intrinsic to medicine. Moreover, this pattern imbues the preclinical years with a feeling of toughness and trial. It is as if they were a necessary evil preceding "real" medical training. The education of contemporary physicians at times seems to recapitulate the history of medicine itself.

Withdrawal, by degrees, from the ignorance of the laity into professional knowledgeableness includes both an extension of knowledge and experience and an extension of uncertainty. It is, as Renee Fox has aptly suggested, a "training for uncertainty"[6] deriving from the disproportion between one's own capacity for knowledge and the amount to be known. It derives further from the fact that often, though by no means always, the scope of reliable information is narrower than the scope of required professional activity. Finally, uncertainty is brought about by the fact that excellence in medical care depends on systematic and impersonal knowledge applied to unique individuals. Patients are unique not because they are exempt from established regularities, but because they, being concrete persons, represent elaborations of both regularities and particular kinds of exceptions. The systematic knowledge that informs their treatment, on the other hand, is inherently abstract.

Medical students enter their training by permission, a permission which in one way or another they have had to earn, partly through academic success. The decision to apply for admission to medical school, itself an important psychological event, typically must be made rather early: medical education now casts its shadow on "premedical" education, since medical education has become incorporated into universities and has ceased to be either an apprenticeship or an enterprise carried on in various proprietary schools. In the main, the commitment to medicine is elusive, representing an investment in effort, time, money, and ease which, in turn, seems to demand that at some later stage one should be able to reap its fruits fully.

As a process, medical education thus combines learning a body of knowledge with techniques for surviving a series of trials and ordeals. Being imposed by teachers upon whom similar trials were imposed earlier, these trials help to justify the students' demands that, in return, all members of each

[6] R. C. Fox, "Training for Uncertainty," in Merton, et al., pp. 207–241.

class be given full permission to enter the ranks of the certified. Willingness to undergo these trials is assumed to be a sign of good faith: one's intention to become a doctor is to be taken seriously.

The intention to commit oneself to a medical life tends, at the beginning, to be accompanied by a disposition toward idealism. This disposition is related to that ambivalence of the laity's image of the medical profession that credits it with capacities it has never claimed, and discredits it with a degree of self-interestedness that escapes fair assessment. Perhaps in a defense against these views, and against their own uncertainties about the motives that actually led them to medical school, medical students often display high hopes concerning their own willingness to help suffering mankind. Initially these hopes come up against the hard requirement of preclinical teaching, often carried out by persons who are not themselves doctors in practice or even in fact. As one persuasive study reports, in the early stage, medical school seems to have little to do with the practice of medicine, which is construed by most students as the treatment of ill people. In spite of the impersonal nature of early medical training, however, idealistic goals are not actually eliminated; rather, they are set aside while the student learns how to get through school.[7] Getting through school transforms aspirations into more realistic conceptions of the hugeness of the medical domain and of the balance of one's own strengths and weaknesses. These perceptions, moreover, are nourished and affected by the judgments and opinions both of faculty members and of one's classmates; between them, faculty and peers form a society that becomes increasingly difficult to leave the longer one stays within it.

[7] H. S. Becker and B. Geer, "The Fate of Idealism in Medical School," *American Sociological Review*, 1958, *23*(1), pp. 50–56.

The Medical Domain

In the course of medical training, the self-images of student physicians and nurses undergo important changes. In the case of nurses, observations in one university and hospital school[8] suggest that in the beginning, nursing is viewed by the trainees as an expression of personal aptitudes and desires. Although nursing is something one has "always wanted to be," at the same time it is also a career that can be suspended for the sake of marriage and children: after all, nursing can serve one in good stead at home, and one can return to it later. As academic preparation gives way to hospital experience and is followed once more by a return to the university, nursing demands the separation of the professional self-image from the private self. Part of oneself has been removed from the laity. But the self has become enlarged, as it were: it is more than what one does professionally. One's profession, with its commitment to neutrality, cannot accommodate all that one is and feels. Furthermore, especially in hospital nursing, what one does is performed within the context of a rather complicated organization that provides a pattern of demands and opportunities into which nurses must fit.

The self-image of medical students, as we have seen, also changes from that of student to that of doctor. This shift is facilitated by increasing clinical contact with patients. In one medical school where contact with patients begins in the first year, it was observed that in two classes of first-year medical students, about one-third already thought of themselves as doctors, not as students, in their dealings with patients; three-quarters believed that patients viewed them as doctors. On the other hand, only 12 per cent thought of themselves as doctors vis-à-vis nurses, and only 8 per cent believed

[8] E. C. Hughes, H. MacGill Hughes, and I. Deutscher, *Twenty Thousand Nurses Tell Their Story.* Philadelphia and Montreal: Lippincott, 1958, especially Chapter 3, "Student Nurses."

Health and Healing

that nurses viewed them in these terms.[9] (To a degree, one's self-image mirrors the images others have of him, and these images are partly known and partly only imagined.) Completion of medical training does not necessarily bring with it a firm self-image as a physician, a fact confirmed by studies in several medical schools.[10] In becoming professional, the self becomes a more complex phenomenon, entering a variety of social relations—with classmates, faculty, patients, and nurses.

In the course of passing examinations and working with patients, aspiring physicians are exposed to a sample of the range of tasks, and the standards applying to those tasks, that define what is expected of them. As expectations confront self-assessments, questions pertaining to self-confidence become important. The student may prefer to use this or that procedure or to deal with this or that type of patient, yet he is asked to assume a role in which he provides uniformly good care for a wide range of patients. The student finds he must meet issues and people as they come to him; he is not free to select his patients by going to them. Such neutrality thrives on confidence. Confidence in one's ability to meet the tasks at hand also enhances one's confidence in being able to deal with uncooperative patients. Relationships with patients are further facilitated when a student is able to proceed without undue affective involvement.

To sum up, medical education, then, like the practice of medicine, is wedded to a body of impersonal knowledge concerning order behind disorder, and to a tradition of artful application of such knowledge. Medicine intervenes, even interferes, preventively or curatively, in the affairs of individuals, at this time or in that place. Medicine is practiced in conditions that change and with changing resources. Mean-

[9] M. J. Huntington, "The Development of a Professional Self-Image," in Merton, et al., Table 21, p. 182.
[10] Huntington, pp. 179–187.

72

while, new generations of physicians and nurses must be trained. They are educated through a complex pattern that in general is guided less by systematic evidence and more by a working consensus forged from both congruent and divergent human experience. In this respect, the process of professional education mirrors one of the basic facts of professional practice: it involves guesswork and risk against a background of demonstrated knowledge.

4

※※※※※※※※※※※※※※※※※※※※※※※

Doctor and
Patient

ᏦᏦᏦᏦᏦᏦᏦᏦᏦᏦᏦᏦᏦᏦᏦᏦᏦᏦᏦᏦᏦᏦ

In Western society, it is believed that ideally the ill should be provided with doctors of their own choice. Once chosen, a doctor who accepts a patient then has the right to expect the latter to be his patient. The patient is not to shop around, comparing diagnoses, costs, and personalities. The encounter between doctor and patient is, after all, potentially or

74

actually part of a relationship; it demands the sharing of private facts, and it is expected to lead to a regime of treatment. The doctor-patient encounter involves a special "contract" through which the doctor's obligation to give of his time is the other side of the patient's obligation to trust, even to depend. Trust and dependency, after all, are characteristic of inclusive, not peripheral, human associations. Finally, doctors are chosen, but need not accept. Unlike nurses in hospitals, they do not offer their services, and they may, for reasons of their own, refuse to become someone's physician. They may impose conditions, some of them economic, others of subtler and more aesthetic character, that govern which patients they will keep and which they will refuse, or even lose.

CHOICE OF PHYSICIAN

So it is in theory; but practice bends and undoes theory, not in defiance of ideals, but rather, because of the variety of ideals and a variety of limiting circumstances that must be reconciled, particularly the following three: First, except in special circumstances, we choose as our physicians people within reasonable reach. We choose, therefore, from a distinctly limited sample of the medical profession. Second, we increasingly often choose doctors from a definite roster of physicians associated with some prepayment plan, to which we belong individually or as families. And third, certain medical conditions, and our own standards of excellence, sometimes require medical treatment that in any one locale (with the exception of certain large cities) can be provided only by very few specialists. These broad and really rather crude selective principles are the major axes of choice; beyond them, a rich pattern of further processes of "discrimination" and selection can be seen.

One might raise the following questions about the choice of a physician: Within any given specialty or general

75

practice, in what sense are doctors not simply interchangeable? Where do their differences lie? To what extent are differences that do not really exist attributed to them? Which of the differences among doctors are simply the result of wishful or fearful positive or negative distortions on the part of patients, or even colleagues? To what extent are clinically relevant differences visible to the laity at all? Our questions give away part of their own answers, and they suggest the genuine difficulties that inquire into this dimension of medical practice encounters.

What is not clinically relevant about a doctor?—that he is a man rather than a woman, old rather than young, soft-spoken rather than of booming voice, Negro rather than white, punctual rather than always late? Surely these things have neither a simple bearing on his medical competence, nor are they simple expressions of it. This list includes quite heterogeneous attributes. Age, for instance, can, though it need not, be the condition of experience. Unless experience be merely the multiplication of the same errors and prejudices through time, it is presumably also an accretion of corrected judgments that can enhance further chances of success and limit future errors. Indeed, a study of women's attitudes about women physicians finds that "experience" counts for much.[1] On the other hand, does skin color or religion influence competence in any simple and consistent way? Clearly, it does not. Yet medical education is not equally available or equally good throughout a society, nor are members of different sectors of a society, for instance Negroes in the United States, equally able to avail themselves of the college preparation necessary for being admitted to and succeeding in medical school.

The choice of a doctor, then, involves a judgment of his competence; and this judgment, which can never be

[1] J. J. Williams, "Patients and Prejudice: Lay Attitudes Toward Women Physicians," *American Journal of Sociology,* 1946, *51*(4), pp. 283–287.

complete, is based on his reputation. This reputation involves judgment concerning his categorical and unique attributes—not only his age, sex, ethnicity, and religion, but also his demeanor or temper. These attributes all affect different people differently. They can act as background principles of selection, or they can become prominent enough to determine selection.

As a result of the whole process of selection, some people remain patients of doctors whom they define as "good" even though they do not, so they say, "like" them; others "like" their doctors even if they have their reservations about their competence. Competence, as we know, varies in kind and degree; and, as medical knowledge does not stand still, the capacity to keep up with the field, even if only selectively, is part of competence. This capacity, however, is limited by many conditions, including the genuine pressures of a good practice, as well as lethargy or self-confidence. Limitations on keeping up also include the legitimate rival claims on a physician's time by the demands of kinship, friendship, and other social relationships.

We must choose our doctor, then, with an eye to what Everett Hughes has called his "auxiliary characteristics."[2] As males, we are likely to wish to be medically treated by men, although there are exceptions to this preference. Also, men are not consistent, for they accept the services of nurses. Women, too, maintain prejudices in favor of male physicians. Generally, in Western cultures, sex and ethnicity, though inherently irrelevant to the professional practice of medicine, become important attributes in patients' choices of doctors and in doctors' choices of medicine as a profession.

In one American study,[3] it became quite clear that not only is the sex of the doctor a matter of importance, but its

[2] E. C. Hughes, *Men and Their Work.* Glencoe, Ill.: Free Press, 1958, p. 103.
[3] Williams, "Patients and Prejudice."

significance is entwined with other considerations. A group of middle-class American women were asked about their attitudes toward female doctors, and it was found that five characteristics of a doctor—experience, sex, ethnicity, religion, and whether or not he or she had been recommended—influenced their choices. It seemed that in America, women (like men) typically prefer to be treated by a male doctor who has had considerable clinical experience, and who is of a religious background similar to one's own. But if women must choose, they prefer to have a doctor who is an experienced woman rather than a very young male physician; and women also prefer a woman to an experienced male Negro doctor.[4]

In other words, the women in this study assumed that there were sex differences in the quality of medical service provided. Why is this? People believe, for instance, that women are more emotional and physically weaker than men, and they would, by this logic, make poor surgeons. Although there are, in fact, not many women surgeons, I suspect that this has much less to do with emotionality or strength than with American images of femininity. Expectations of the feminine woman tend to rule out the kind of disciplined aggressiveness, endurance, and control generally required in surgery. Surgery also demands the assumption of responsibility and authority under socially isolated conditions, again, out of keeping with the image of a feminine woman, whose area of authority is limited to the young.

Presumably, if it were known that women are markedly disinclined to go to female physicians, this knowledge would reduce the eagerness of women to enter medical schools and so to enlist in the battles of a professional minority. One of the specialties that female physicians enter is pediatrics; however, in the future there will probably be more women physicians of

[4] Williams, p. 287.

all kinds, as the integration of women into the professional world increases.

Women are reluctant to consult doctors of different ethnic backgrounds, and explanations for it differ. Prejudice against women doctors may be acknowledged as silly, and prejudice against Negro doctors, or doctors representing other ethnic or religious minorities, may be clearly undemocratic, yet such sentiments affect people's actions. It would seem, though, that a single contact with a woman physician, whether satisfactory or not, is likely to lead to a new view of women doctors. A single contact with a member of an ethnic or racial minority is more likely to be "dismissed as the 'exception that proves the rule' when it does not conform to expectations."[5]

To summarize, women appear to balance their preferences for physicians in the following ways: their first choice is for experienced, male doctors, recommended to them by others, and whose religious faith is like their own. Anything different, in the eyes of most, is a drawback. However, if the choice involves experience versus the appropriate faith and sex, experience wins.

To discuss the laity's choice of doctors is to consider, as well, the profession's selection of its members. In my account of medical education I suggested how the licensing of medical practitioners gives to medical schools a final monopoly for the supply of the doctors from whom, subsequently, the population can choose. Doctors also choose, if only by determining the specialty they prefer to practice in and the locale in which they wish to work. Thus, between the actions of medical schools and the preferences of individual doctors, patients in any particular community are provided with a specifically limited array of physicians among whom they can make their complex choices.

[5] Williams, p. 287.

Health and Healing

Illness is part of the impersonal order of nature. All animals sicken and so die; even cure, considered as restoration, is not confined to human orders. We speak of *vis mediatrix naturae,* the "curative power of nature." Our concern here, however, is with illness among human beings who are conscious of each other's presence. For them, and for those who observe them, illness is one of several modes of plight. In our society, clinical encounters are one kind of arrangement expected to help in the resolution of those plights that we attribute to illness, and they share elements with other human encounters. Getting advice, seeing a doctor, being counseled by a priest, putting one's affairs into the hands of a lawyer, all have both common themes and variations on those themes.

Clinical arrangements are the concrete social instruments for the restitution or enhancement of a disordered state of affairs.[6] Typically, clinical encounters take place between two people, and in privacy, although this pattern is not universal. Curing can take place in public; it can even require public confession. But curing does, in some sense, involve the inspection of a particular person, and persons have both private and public aspects, the private side being emphasized in most healing arrangements. Our society goes a long way in withdrawing those to be cured from their ordinary milieu, at least for certain procedures. To be sure, we sustain a variety of arrangements in this regard. Operations are an encounter between more than two people, and medical examinations often take place in the presence of a third person. Even psychotherapy, an attempt at exploring private history as well as present dilemmas, can take place with the aid of groups. Still, we associate cure with a fiduciary relationship: someone

[6] E. H. Erikson, "The Nature of Clinical Evidence," *Daedalus,* 1958, 87.(4), pp. 65–87.

80

is in need of help, someone else is in a position to provide help.

The clinical encounter, in other words, implies a certain kind of contract: "In exchange for a fee, and for information revealed in confidence, the physician promises to act for the benefit of the individual patient, within the ethos of the profession."[7] Typically, the patient can be anybody; but the doctor, being a qualified person, cannot just be anybody. The clinical encounter, therefore, is asymmetrical and implies inequality, and therefore provides an opportunity for the exploitation of helplessness. Because of this asymmetry, clinical encounters demand provisions that ensure that doctors are not only doing their best, but also are not doing any avoidable harm.

Physicians may have to increase the plight of their patients temporarily, however, in order to help them, and the patients, whether of their own accord or under various kinds of duress, must surrender much of their personal inviolability to a qualified person who does not, in turn, surrender his. Curers, whatever their past, are presumed to be themselves well enough to cure. They participate in the patient's disclosures and inspect his condition, but at a distance, and so the asymmetry is compounded.

Doctors, furthermore, see more than they are told, for they listen and observe with the help of their special knowledge. Such knowledge entails a mode of thinking both about the body of the patient and about the "whole patient." To think about the latter, however, is to think about oneself as well, for the whole patient is only revealed through his relationship to the doctor. The clinical encounter involves the assessment of another who both actively complains and passively offers himself for inspection; it involves the assembling of fragments into both a diagnosis and a prognosis for the sake of selecting a method of treatment.

[7] Erikson, p. 66.

Health and Healing

The clinician not only bridges the spheres of the well and the ill, but he also links the past to the present for the sake of the future. He takes a history; he wrestles with what is relevant. He recognizes that different states of sickness are of different penetrability at his level of knowledge, and that the subjective complaints of a patient, although necessary, are often not sufficient to indicate the cure. The physician intervenes, but he does so with the cooperation and even help of the patient. The patient learns modes of observation that in part he can, and at times he must, appropriate to himself. Thus, as he becomes a case for another, he also becomes one for himself.

We know that such a coordinated process depends upon special social arrangements. We know that these very arrangements may, in themselves, be part of the reason for some restitutive success. The clinical encounter, especially in Western society, provides a contrast to the usual succession of situations in which adults are involved day by day. It is, in some respects, reminiscent of childhood and domesticity. Only in the context of domesticity are we accustomed to display that conjunction of physical nakedness and social dependency that are potentially involved in cure.

In the clinical encounter, we must lay ourselves bare and acknowledge our relative helplessness and deprivation; even the occasion for doing so constitutes a deprivation, for we have been interrupted by illness. Such an interruption may become the occasion for inner or outer developments that could otherwise not have occurred and that may ultimately be to our benefit. But this is another story.

We move into clinical encounters, precisely because by our own or someone else's account we have become insufficient. When we are in an emotional plight or have become mentally ill, it may well be, as Lévi-Strauss suggests, that our impasse consists in not finding the world sufficiently textured for

the excessive richness that is within us.[8] In contrast, the plight
of the "normally," that is, physically, ill person is to find
sufficient meaning in a world that is temporarily too complex
for him. In such an impasse we come to require some authority.

It is clear that only a particular configuration of expectations on the part of both doctor and patient will allow
cure to proceed, and will keep within limits the possible
distortion of perspectives inherent in the crisis of illness. This
crisis, as we have seen, is met by doctors and nurses with
technical knowledge and disciplined subjectivity, which, in
combination, lead to both the taking and the making of a
case history. Thus is established the regime of cure.

As a rule, this kind of regime cannot be set up between
friends, but requires a "professional relationship." It can,
however, be done under varying conditions of privacy or
publicity, whenever doctor and patient constitute a nexus in
which each has circumscribed responsibilities. The emotionality
of one is balanced by the steadiness of the other, and the self-
centeredness of the patient is limited by the curer's concern
with his welfare. This delicate balance demands trust, obedience, and a kind of intimacy; but despite all this, the curer
remains an outsider to whom a fee is due.

On this ground plan of a curing relationship, various
elaborations are possible. In the West, we have gone further
than most societies in associating medical care with confidentiality and with those technical aids that can render the
physician relatively independent of his own subjective assess-
ments. We have sought to reduce the magical element in
therapy. We have arranged clinical encounters so that they
make possible the confrontation of the kinds of facts, which, if

[8] See C. Lévi-Strauss, *Anthropologie Structurale*. Paris,
Librairie Plon, 1958, Chapter IX. There has just appeared an
English translation by C. Jacobson and B. G. Schoepf, *Structural
Anthropology*. New York, Basic Books, 1963, pp. 167–185.

announced elsewhere, might lead to ridicule or punishment. We have come to demand that for all their ties with society and its moralities, the medical fraternity and the professions allied with it represent an order of ethical neutrality. In the confines of this neutrality we, the patients, can then have the courage to see ourselves as less than we might want to be. We can even extend our experience of illness to include a new awareness of ourselves as an assemblage of bodily parts.

Cure, as a form of restoration or rebirth, therefore, can involve some temporary suspension of awareness of oneself as person. In this, it resembles sleep. But cure also involves work or discipline. We then speak of the "course" that treatment takes. This course involves people who have their being in other spheres of life than clinical encounters. Much of what goes into medical practice involves talk, discussion, mutual interpretation, the exercise of authority, and the giving of orders. Doctors exert influence and represent a style of thought. By inference they represent a style of life. They make demands on patients. The latter, in turn, try to give them what they want, at least in some measure.

Professional training, and subsequent professional income, can remove doctors from many of the spheres from which their patients come. In some orderly fashion they are less than equidistant from the patients or their practice, for they share a style of life with some and quite obviously not with others. Their training, moreover, especially in North America, tends to have crowded out any extended opportunities for considering the various social patterns into which the illnesses of their patients fall. We should not be surprised, therefore, if certain sectors of the population stay away from medical care even when such care is made available without direct cost, because they feel the great distance between themselves and the medical world, and cannot risk the clinical encounter.

84

5

$\approx$

Cost of Medical Care

$\approx$

Whatever its benefits, illness, once it is more than slight and fleeting, yields a variety of costs. Some seem in the main to be "economic": loss of time, of income, of accomplishment. Illness also demands payment of a variety of medical costs, including insurance against greater costs. The latter expenditure we call health insurance, an ambiguous expression covering a variety of schemes that represent, not the possibility of ensuring one's health, but an attempt at reducing the concentration—and to a lesser extent, the absolute amount—of medical expenditure. Insurance is an attempt at dissociating the quality of medical care from too simple a relation to a patient's ability to pay. We are still in search of ways of supplying doctors, hospitals, nurses, medication, and care in relation to the conditions of health of a society, rather than in relation to its wealth.

COSTS FOR THE PATIENT

If we confine ourselves to the United States and to the last twenty years, it is quite clear that private expenditures for medical care and voluntary health insurance have risen steadily. In 1953 they amounted to about 10.2 billion dollars, by 1958 to about 16.2 billion dollars.[1] To put it in the form of an average, which hides many important differences, in 1957 a person would spend about $5 out of every $100 on matters of health, disease, and death; $29 on food; $9 on clothing; $33 on housing and the running of his home; and $11 on transportation.[2] In 1929, he would have spent just about the same for medical expenses, more for clothes and less for food, more on his house, and less for travel.

If we use the consumer price index, the cost of medical care has steadily risen, but remains unequal for different parts of the country. In 1963, using averages again, a general practitioner in Vancouver, Canada, would charge about $11.25 for a first office visit with complete examination; in California, $10.00; and in Seattle, Washington, $7.50.[3] In studying the

[1] O. W. Anderson, et al., "Family Expenditure Patterns for Personal Health Services," *HIF Research Series 14*, 1960, Table 1, p. 3.
[2] H. J. Greenfield and O. W. Anderson, "The Medical Care Price Index," *HIF Research Series*, 1959, 7, Table 1, p. 2.
[3] Figures drawn from various fee schedules as listed in *The Vancouver Sun*, December 14, 1963, p. 22.

expenditures of farmers in Vermont from 1800 until 1940, and in charting their ups and downs, we see an uninterrupted and steady ascent of physicians' fees. These hardly even vary in their increments from one year to the next, but slowly and regularly climb higher.[4]

There are, of course, reasons for this climb. The cost of medical care, including medical training, is greater, especially when one comes to expect uniformly good university education, a widespread enterprise of medical research, modern hospital accommodation, and the maintenance of a private system of medical care within the context of an aging population with increasing numbers of chronically ill people. In England, between 1940 and 1954, the total net cost of the national health service, a public system of medicine, also went up, yet, as a proportion of the "gross national product," the cost of the English health service in fact went down during that period. In the ten years between 1940 and 1950, 8 of every 100 pounds were involved in the health service; in 1953–1954, the percentage dropped to 3.4.[5]

ECONOMY OF HEALTH AND ILLNESS

Medical economics is a highly specialized field. It is also the battleground for the debate over the relative merits of different forms of economic arrangements for the provision of and recompense for medical services, in either the narrower or wider sense of that term. The many technicalities of the debate on where the fiscal responsibility for medical care lies clearly must not concern us here; they involve the question of prepayment, by a large or small population, for a changing population of illnesses, accidents, and medical needs. Illness,

[4] H. J. Greenfield and O. W. Anderson, "The Medical Care Price Index," *HIF Research Series 7,* 1959, Chart I and pp. 11ff.

[5] H. Eckstein, *The English Health Service.* Cambridge: Harvard University Press, 1958, Table 5 and pp. 217–221.

as we know, is unequally distributed through a population. It is, as well, subject to a variety of changes. Some of the latter are predictable, some are not. In addition, the state of health of a society, even under the most modern of conditions, is still subject to a variety of unexpected contingencies, such as epidemics, or the by-products of accidents in connection with such enterprises as atomic energy projects, and technical failures, which include the use of faulty vaccines. Part of the institutional arrangement of medical care must provide for the possibility of such contingencies. (Furthermore, specific programs of prevention or restitution cannot exhaust the medical domain of health. Part of it, especially public health, has obligations similar to the purposes and activities of fire departments.)

Often the terms of the debate over the best financial and organizational forms for medical care becloud the issues involved. Much is made, as we have said, of the doctor-patient relationship, while the character of that relation remains, perhaps deliberately, vague. Furthermore, there are probably several different kinds of such relationships, all compatible with "good" or "successful" patterns of prevention or therapy. As we know from the English case, government sponsorship of an inclusive, yet ultimately voluntary, health service in no way needs to interfere with the possibilities of certain kinds of doctor-patient relations, including the free choice of doctor and patient of one another.

As we have said, such choice is never absolutely free even under the least regulated of medical patterns. Doctors are never equally good or equally accessible or equally distributed over the population. Nor is a totally unregulated medical practice, absolutely divorced from the nonmedical agencies of government and law, even conceivable. The debate, then, concerns the kind and mode of regulation, not the presence or absence of it; it concerns the scope that private insurance and prepayment schemes should have in relation to schemes sponsored by government or large-scale corporate enterprises such as trade unions. The debate concerns the desirable balance among the following valued activities: maximizing a population's health through medical care; maintaining individual freedom of choice of specialty, location, and clientele on the part of the doctor; allowing patients to choose their doctor; enhancing the scope and quality of medical education and research; matching the professional resources of a country with the range of its human requirements; and fitting one tradition of excellence to a complicated, divided, and divergent pattern of human interaction.

The debate also involves questions of economy and efficiency. These terms must, however, receive specially adapted meanings when one deals not with the production of a useful thing like soap, but with the administration of a useful preventive service like a vaccination program to successive generations of school children. Economy and efficiency cannot be excluded from the arrangements, private and public, that govern the management of human plight. How to count cost in the context of plight is, however, another matter. Such an accounting is different under conditions where one is simply concerned with maximizing profits and minimizing losses. Finally, of course, the economy of health and illness looks rather different from the different points of view of those involved. "The best possible" provision of care is surely one thing when considered from the point of view of doctors, another when discussed by hospital administrators, a third when debated by an upper-class, middle-aged lady from Philadelphia, and a fourth when considered by an immigrant farm laborer. This point is both easily overlooked and easily overstressed. Indeed, one of the issues here has been precisely the question: what is good medical practice? What costs are we incurring for the sake of what gains?

Health and Healing

Let us add at least some details to suggest the dimensions of the problem of social cost. Studies of the economics of mental illness distinguish between direct and indirect costs.[6] The former refers to actual dollar expenditures for mental illness, including the amount spent by government, by a variety of private philanthropies, and by individuals on the care, cure, and prevention of mental illness. The latter is a very inclusive expression. Indirect cost refers to the actual economic loss in dollars or work years that, as a society, we sustain because part of society is ill. In the case of mental health care in the United States, that part is estimated to be about 6 per cent of the population. The direct costs of mental illness are over 1.7 billion dollars a year.

This estimate is conservative. If one adds to direct costs, indirect cost, which is clearly a more elusive quantity, the total bill comes to about 2.4 billion dollars per year for mental illness. It may be that in increasing the direct costs, that is, in spending more money for the care and prevention of this illness as of any other illness, we will eventually reduce the indirect cost. The better the quality of medical care, however, the more the public may want to make use of it, and the higher the costs will be. There is probably no simple relation between expenditure now and reduction of expenditure later. It is, however, more than likely that we shall save ourselves expenditures in the future by not saving certain expenditures now.

Costs in this context are only in part precisely measurable. Besides, although the study from which I have taken my facts does not specifically mention this, one person's expenditure is always another person's income. The question

[6] R. Fein, *Economics of Mental Health,* Joint Commission on Mental Health and Illness, Monograph Series No. 2. New York: Basic Books, 1958.

90

becomes: what should and what can a society spend on any illness, or on all illnesses together? To a degree it has no choice. It will pay in one way or another for the illnesses that come and do not quickly leave, through loss of time and persons or through an accumulation of pain and frustration that hampers the flow of satisfactions on which the continuity of life depends. To put it in the form of the classic dilemma: Given the scarcity of human resources, how should they be distributed? How much should go to education and how much to health and how much to national security? To what extent, moreover, should any part of this dilemma be left to individual resolution?

Each country, in fact, reveals its own solution to this dilemma in what actually occurs. But what occurs is not immutable. Money could be spent differently, because the enterprise of promoting health or reducing illness calls for various choices. The general debate over the relative roles of different levels of government within the medical domain is only one such issue of choice. Another issue arises precisely from the success of the medical domain itself. We have reduced infant mortality, and thus we have secured the chance of keeping alive a wide range of persons with very unequal vulnerabilities for subsequent debilities, all of them, within limits, equally free to reproduce. This may yield us considerable future cost, yet it may well be worth it, especially if such cost is considered the sweet and bitter fruit of personal freedom.

It seems to be true, in the United States at least, that the lower a family's income, the greater is the percentage of that income laid out for personal health services. It is also true that a large number of American families are in debt to hospitals, physicians, and dentists. The Hippocratic enjoinder for the healer to heal the poor in disregard of his financial inability is obviously not workable, nor is the older system of making the rich pay for the free service that their doctors give to the poor. There may be justice in the latter pattern, for the skills of doctors were often developed with the help of clinical experiences in outpatient departments, or at clinics held at the bedsides of indigent patients in public wards. It was, however, the middle groups between the rich and the indigent that then suffered the most under medical bills. Now it is the older groups of the population, for whom insurance is more difficult or expensive, who constitute one of the most difficult problems for medical economics. Ironically, these old people represent the success of the medical domain because many of them have been cured of illnesses that once would have ended their lives.

PHYSICIAN'S FINANCIAL ARRANGEMENT

An intimate aspect of medical economics, especially in the absence of impersonal methods of prepayment or insurance, is the physician's own financial management. Doctors often surround themselves with a variety of services, like collecting agencies and telephone answering services. On occasion, they must face the problem of collecting their bills, and they must keep books and financial records themselves or else pay someone to do so for them.

What are the precise ways in which such economic arrangements affect specific doctor-patient relations? This issue is full of belief and empty of fact. Modes of payment do not flourish by themselves; they are, in turn, part of a wider set of arrangements. Local medical societies, for instance, help to set scales and fees which are used as broad guides by individual practitioners whose patients may compare both the care they are receiving and the price they are paying with the parallel experiences of others.

Because illness happens to one and is, presumably, not sought, it seems a double misfortune to both suffer it and to have to pay a price for its cure. Logically this may seem specious, especially as what is being paid for is presumably not illness but the restoration of health. Health, surely, like wealth, esteem, or some specific accomplishments, is an object of men's wants, and as such it is caught in the calculus of income and expenditure. Yet health is not a specific accomplishment and may, for all we know, be attainable only indirectly. We may have to think of our medical bills primarily in terms of specific and definite interventions intended to prevent illness or undo its occurrence.

The pain and deprivation of illness are themselves separable from the cost in dollars of medical care. The latter cost is presumably less than the former, especially if we consider how uncured illness radiates. Contagion, furthermore, is only one form of such radiation, and probably not the most serious.

Illness, in its genuine or feigned appearances, can, as we have argued, constitute a form of withdrawal from ordinary obligations. It may also be an avenue toward the assumption of extraordinary or interstitial obligations. Leaving aside this complication, and leaving aside also the fact that certain chronically yet not seriously ill persons may perform very important functions within certain social circles, illness does constitute a burden on the well and a reduction of the vitality available for the pursuit of the ends for which people live. The medical domain disperses this burden. Its efforts clearly justify recompense, but such recompense must combine income with honor.

A differentiated and effective medical domain requires economic resources in large proportions. Moreover, it requires them for the maintenance of institutions, notably hospitals, which cannot as a rule be financed simply through the income from patients. Furthermore, some medical enterprises, especially research institutes, have no direct and specific consumers.

Others, like medical schools, require sums far in excess of the economic abilities of students and their families. Specific doctor-patient relations and their financial settlements are thus part of a wider economic web. This fact strengthens the argument of those who would urge that payment for clinical encounters come from more impersonal, collective, or public sources. Moreover, as a professional person, a doctor is presumably less governed than many others by an obvious and announced interest in making money or profits.

The situation is further complicated by the fact that the doctor wants not only money from his patients; he demands acceptance from them. He must do things for and to them, which helps obscure the importance of the patient's ability to pay and the physician's dependence on this ability. In view of this economic asymmetry, which runs counter to the professional asymmetry that gives the doctor authority over the patient, we should not be surprised that doctors experience difficulties in collecting their fees. Such difficulties, though by no means unique to physicians, assume characteristic forms in the medical domain. We should perhaps not be surprised that fees, the symbols of the value of medical care, are high.

In ordinary office practice, it is probably the rule that cash payment to the doctor by the patient after each consultation tends not to be the ideal way of settling the question of the doctor's and the patient's dependence on one another. To a degree, the method of sending bills is a matter of tradition and circumstances, including social class, mobility and travel, and rural-urban differences. The ideal is to segregate economic transactions from professional consultations or specific services. Such segregation can involve the use of third parties—a nurse, a secretary, or an insurance firm. The latter introduces further complications: whereas the nurse and secretary are employed by the physician himself, prepaid medical schemes or collective health services contain the doctor and his patients in wider and very specific agreements.

Given the segregation of the economic from the technical and social components of the relations between doctors or institutions and their patients, the economic component stands a chance of falling between various extremes. It can, in its simplest form, be a matter settled between doctor and patient: the former charges a fee, the latter pays. Bargaining is likely to be frowned upon, though patients may ask for an opportunity to spread their payments. In the case of dentistry, in America and Canada at least, the total bill usually can be known after the first consultation and can thus become subject to various arrangements. At another extreme, as in Russia, the majority of doctors, especially the young ones, draw a salary or are paid fees for services from funds not directly collected from patients, but indirectly collected from the whole population.

Direct settlement between doctors and patients is subject to the flexibilities of a sliding scale, and is affected by local customs and conditions. The doctor's fees, moreover, may be set in terms of the management of some particular event, such as pregnancy and postpartum care, regardless of the volume of work entailed, or it may be a function of the amount of time and effort entailed in the cure of some specific ailment.

Direct settlement represents, it is argued, the maximum of freedom, or control, in the relation between doctor and patient. Under its rule, both are free from external interference. A just and discriminating analysis of this assumption is at the moment frustrated by the absence of the necessary dispassionate information. We have already suggested that the precise effects of specific economic arrangements on the relations between doctors and patients are hard to gauge because they are subtle and often elusive. Nor is it conclusively clear what kinds of doctor-patient relations have what kinds of effects on cure, since cure is, except in the simplest of ailments, a more ambiguous phenomenon than might first appear. It is clear, however, from the evidence available from the American experience with prepaid schemes and English experiences with the National Health Service,[7] that the source and mode of remuneration of a doctor are within wide limits independent of the maintenance of the order of freedom classically considered as necessary for the mutual trust and concern that marks the encounters between doctors and patients.

The doctor's and patient's free choice of one another is never absolute, even under the most private and least public of arrangements. Even a national health scheme may not necessarily, as is sometimes alleged, turn a free profession into a civil service. It can become a joint venture, in which the medical profession retains virtually complete control over the substance of its work, patients retain the right to choose the doctor whom they wish, and the government, as third party, concentrates on providing funds and facilities. Under such an arrangement, the various elements of medical practice— economic, technical, social, and personal—cease to be confounded. Such a venture would directly control specific physicians only through setting limits to the total number of patients they might have on their books, and through demanding certain kinds of information from them. If these demands led to paper work, this would not be incompatible with the explicit standards of Western medicine.

Under certain economic arrangements, some doctors become employees of the state. This arrangement raises dilemmas, and offends some, if by no means all, of the values implicit in the democratic tradition. In such cases, however,

[7] Cf. O. W. Anderson and P. B. Sheatsley, "Comprehensive Medical Insurance," *HIF Research Series 9,* 1959, and H. Eckstein, *The English Health Service.* Cambridge: Harvard University Press, 1958.

medical-economic arrangements are simply an expression of a different general philosophy of individual freedom and the role of the state, rather than an intrinsic difference in the practice of medicine.

We must then distinguish the source and mode of a doctor's income from the order of freedom and constraint under which he works. Third parties may actually enhance his freedom, whereas the absence of collective arrangements may reduce it. Besides, doctors do not have merely a series of discrete and specific patients. They have a practice, and in it they depend on a whole web of other social arrangements to which, in turn, they themselves contribute.

We have learned from the Russians that the employment of doctors by agencies of a state can force doctors into the dilemma of having to keep in mind both the requirements of society and the requirements of their own patients. We know, for example, that Russian doctors are under pressure to make sharp distinctions between malingering and genuine illness. They are expected to give the former as little encouragement as possible so that a maximum amount of energy is available for the demands of the economy.[8] In the West we would reject such a system in the name of a very different conception of the rights of individuals, the proper role of government, and freedom for the professions.

In spite of our repudiation of the Russian way, we, too, use the free professions in the service of large institutional arrangements, military and industrial, educational and religious. We also require a fair number of professional people to exercise their competence within the conditions of bureaucratic employment. This is especially true of public health officers,

[8] M. G. Field, *Doctor and Patient in Soviet Russia.* Cambridge: Harvard University Press, 1957, especially Chapter 9, "To certify or not to certify: The Physician's Dilemma," pp. 146–180.

psychiatrists working in public mental hospitals, and the medical services provided for the Veterans Administration. We also know that creative scientific research and clinical investigation are sustained by professional people on the staffs of the federal government's National Institutes of Health.

Certain financial arrangements associated with the use of prepayment and third parties can, directly or unintentionally, come to exert pressures that affect clinical practices. Sometimes surgical procedures are affected this way. In other words, third parties can be used in quite different ways, only some of which are wholly compatible with that mode of interrelation between doctor and patient that the former, if not the latter, demands. On the one hand, the complete segregation of economic transactions can enhance those aspects of the clinical encounter that involve the experience of intimacy, trust, confidentiality, and personal concern, which, in our society, are typically removed from the worldly considerations of economic calculation. On the other hand, even the most personal of relations inevitably involves economic resources even if these are simply a matter of the allocation of time. It is also true that professional aid requires distance, and money can be a convenient symbol for distance.

The payment for medical services, in other words, presents some characteristic difficulties that separate this settlement of debt from the settlements of other debts. Like works of art, the services of a doctor are not easily measurable, they are sought rather than offered, and their evaluation exceeds the layman's judgment. We would expect, then, that doctors would have least trouble in collecting their bills when they provide preventive or pediatric services, because the more tangible and meaningful the medical service becomes, the easier it seems to secure payment for it. Services involving inoculation and other routine procedures, especially when provided to children, have the fiscal advantage of being less expensive and the psychological advantage of being more predictable. Serious illnesses, in contrast, come unexpectedly, and as a shock for which a charge seems the addition of insult to injury. In a measure, then, the collecting of accounts becomes more difficult as the illness becomes more serious; if the doctor has only recently acquired the patient to whom he must send bills, it may be more difficult still.

Finally, direct payment may help in the development and expression of that sense of ownership—implied by the expression "my doctor"—that tends to go with professional bonds. Moreover, as Freud argued in connection with psychotherapy, the attempt to cure implies a serious contract between healer and patient, which in turn requires its symbols of cost and sacrifice.

The success of the English Health Service, the Canadian Provincial-Federal agreements concerning hospital insurance, and the continuous growth of group practice throughout the Western world, all show that within rather wide limits the same professional relation, binding healers and patients, can flourish under different economic arrangements.

Ultimately, any society must face the economic question, what is the best distribution of its medical resources, given the distribution of demands for these resources? Illness and cure are both created from the materials of nature within the order of society. (Some illnesses, even, are the very results of cure.)

We have a choice. We can recognize explicitly the relationships among illness, health, and the social order, or we can leave them implicitly understood. We can choose the uncoordinated patterns of a maximum of private enterprise, with its greater freedom for at least some individuals, or the more coordinated pattern of a planned mixture of private and public arrangements, with its greater control but greater equity. We are not entirely free in our choice, however, because

Health and Healing

we do not start from scratch. We are, for instance, the bene-factors of a medical domain that has traditionally distributed its preventive resources only when provided with organized institutional methods for distributing them. We are also members of a society in which we live so close to so many people that our health and others' are intimately interconnected. These legacies from the past and others like them constrain the choices we can make in the future.

We have banished the grosser epidemics only because we have come to expect and accept an obvious and subtle web of public health measures and legislative devices. In spite of our gains, the balance between public and private medicine must continue to be negotiated, especially if we are to recruit able and reliable people for the medical profession, reward them with that sense of calling and honor that is characteristic of the older professions, and still provide ourselves with a pattern of medical services that is not found wanting when its equality, efficiency, technical competence, and genuine compassion are all assessed.

6

Cure Beyond the Medical Domain

$\mathbb{C}$uring can never be wholly a professional monopoly, and in this it differs from some of the activities of
other professions, such as litigation. Although litigation, like
curing, is part of the professional domain of a specific professional tradition, at least in industrialized societies, it involves
a complete monopoly by agencies of the state and cannot be

101

carried on outside the courts. Settlements out of court are a different matter, being contracts, not litigation. In other words, some activities of the legal profession are wholly a professional concern; however, no aspect of cure is wholly medical.

The sphere of activities in which the nonprofessional forms of curing exist, however, is not of one piece. At a minimum, we should distinguish between specialized alternatives to the official tradition of professional medical practice, such as Christian Science; marginal professional activities such as chiropractic; folk medicine; and quackery.

We are well aware that these distinctions are relative, and that this relativity is compounded by the ambiguity of definition that attends them all. We know from the domain of religion that the dogma of today can be the heresy of yesterday, or tomorrow. Similarly, the emphasis placed by Christian Science on the emotional or spiritual dimensions of illness, which was for so long ridiculed, has gained ascendancy once more. The degree of professional legitimacy of cure through faith that attends modern psychosomatic medicine could hardly have been foreseen in the middle of the nineteenth century.

CHIROPRACTIC

Throughout the world, there are about thirty thousand chiropractors, most of them active in the United States and Canada, and a majority of these practicing in the middle and far West. In calling these chiropractors marginally professional, I do not make any invidious implication. They are professional because they are licensed, and they are involved in the application of a specialized body of knowledge that is taught in specific and regulated institutions requiring definite amounts of time before the trainees are allowed to practice and to develop a clientele. The legal status of this particular group of practitioners is not uniform throughout the United States, however, and their distribution is not uniform.

Cure Beyond the Medical Domain

My justification for concentrating on chiropractors is that Walter Wardwell's excellent study of this group is available.[1] It remains to be seen to what extent the implications of this study's findings can also apply to such other marginal medical professions as chiropodists, osteopaths, and the like.

There are two varieties of chiropractic, represented by two national associations—the National Chiropractic Association, which in 1951 had some 7,700 members, and the International Chiropractors' Association, which at the same time had about 3,500 members. The latter association was more orthodox, and held the view that chiropractors should limit themselves to spinal manipulations. The National Association was a "mixer" organization, and went beyond the International group in sanctioning the use of heat, light, air, water, exercise, and diet in therapy. Members of the International organization looked upon members of the National one as having sold out to the pressures of the medical profession.

The majority of chiropractors come from the less privileged social positions, and the acquisition of chiropractic skills means upward mobility for them. If income is a measure of prestige, chiropractors are comparable to dentists, optometrists, and chiropodists. Many chiropractors are, of course, motivated by a genuine desire to aid the sick, and it is impossible to tell how many of them would have preferred medical school but were financially unable to enter it. If these practitioners are motivated alike by a wish to succeed and a wish to minister to the ill, they do not differ markedly from medical doctors. They do differ in the scope of their ultimate training and in their professional competence, which, although licensed, is fairly intimately related to a very specific theory of illness. This theory, incidentally, would attribute a great deal of

[1] W. I. Wardwell, "A Marginal Professional Role: The Chiropractor," in E. G. Jaco (Ed.), *Patients, Physicians, and Illness.* Glencoe, Ill.: Free Press, 1958, pp. 421–433.

103

human suffering to the status of the human spine, the proper manipulation of which becomes a preferred method of cure and the primary claim to professional standing among fellow chiropractors. If we call this claim marginal, it is partly because of the attitude of the medical profession, which has, in conjunction with the licensing bodies, helped to limit the scope of practice of this group.

Being legally limited in the scope of his medical practice, the chiropractor, though often disapproved by professional medical bodies, tends, nevertheless, to become in some way associated with physicians because he must, on occasion, refer patients to them. Given the status of chiropractic, it is not surprising to find that, unlike the medical profession, it does tend to engage in a certain amount of advertising and soliciting. In spite of all the limitations suggested, the relations between chiropractors and their clients are not too different from the relationship between physicians and their patients, and they are not, surprisingly, more informal and less professional.

Taking chiropractors as representatives of a wider range of marginal professional roles, we can look at their clientele for some clues to their existence. If these marginal roles are not entirely generated by the limitations of the medical domain itself, they are, in a measure at least, maintained by it. More chiropractic patients, for instance, seem to come from the lower rather than the upper classes, and many patients come for treatment as a last resort after medical men have failed to cure them. Many of the patients of chiropractors have had long and unsuccessful histories of contact with the established medical profession. The clientele, moreover, seems to contain a fair proportion of hypochondriacs and neurotics, who are likely to be dissatisfied with orthodox medical treatment, especially when such treatment is not oriented to psychological issues. As a group, these patients are in search of hope, help, a certain amount of personal contact with their doctors, and the relatively simple explanations for a fairly wide range of disorders that the chiropractor is willing to provide. They especially want explanations for emotional disturbances that make the causes of their plight palpable. Repeated visits for treatment by massage or manipulation provide an order of intimacy that more orthodox and conventional practice, at least in the eyes of these patients, seems to lack. We should not be surprised, then, that the medical profession disapproves of chiropractic while at the same time individual doctors maintain a variety of relations with it.

The success of chiropractors serves the medical domain by providing it with an opportunity to reassess the scope and direction of its own practices. Such a reassessment involves, among other matters, this persistent question: How can the inculcation of standards of excellence during a long medical training be made compatible with the maintenance or development of understanding for segments of the population whose education and style of life are removed from the manner and style of life of practicing doctors? The chiropractor, who is probably more patient-oriented than many physicians, does undoubtedly help fill a vacuum created by the doctor's trained incapacity to understand certain patients. He offers a helpful intimacy that is professional in that it is not reciprocal and does not extend the patient's obligations, and he represents simple solutions that serve to express the doubts of patients about the sufficiency or even necessity of established medical practice.

If the medical profession is seriously concerned with reducing the numbers of marginal professionals, it will be most successful if it tries to incorporate the advantages of these practices into its own tradition. Such incorporation may be seen by some as an insult to the standards of excellence from which the medical practitioner derives a sense of identity and worth. Nevertheless, if family practitioners are to become reestablished on a higher plane of esteem than the rapid growth of specialization has until recently allowed, they will also, presumably, come to incorporate a more distinct concern with the elusive, human issues surrounding the particular complaints of their patients. Such a concern might reduce the number of dissatisfied patients who, not wishing to give up hope, seek out alternative helpers. If doctors had a greater concern with the human aspects of medicine, it would be possible for those ill people with whom present-day physicians can find nothing particularly wrong, but who nevertheless define themselves as ill, to remain under ordinary medical care without being defined as malingerers.

Besides providing havens for difficult patients, marginal professions also suggest possible additions to traditional medical practice by pointing up that in its present form medicine fails to acknowledge adequately those aspects of illness that the marginal profession makes into its own specialty.

The tension between legitimate and marginal professional practices places limits on the conservatism that accompanies all professional activity. The history of medicine suggests that, until recently, the marriage of medicine to the ever-changing resources of science is not enough for the maintenance of a continuous revision of actual practices because specific human practices involving the management of the plight of other people are always more than a matter of scientific knowledge.

Whereas the laity demands simple and quick solutions to minimize the loss and deprivation that illness can easily entail, the medical profession in its attachment to standards of excellence, must reject the demand that it take the simplest or quickest or cheapest way out. Rigid perfectionism, however, only enhances malpractice, marginal professional activity, and quackery.

Cure Beyond the Medical Domain

We can easily imagine that the existence of marginal professional roles provides opportunities for a sense of martyrdom, especially in those states where chiropractors are not licensed. Such martyrdom feeds on a sense of persecution. Marginal professionals often tend to see such persecution as coming not from the medical profession as a whole, but from a small group of politically powerful individuals within the formal structure of the profession. Consequently, such practitioners develop a sense of righteousness and rightness and become all the more convinced of their philosophy. Even where chiropractic does not succeed, for instance, the principles of chiropractic are not questioned, because they are perceived almost as a sacred truth that provides certainty and does not fail. Any failure is ascribed not to the cure but to the curer, who will be expected to apply the principle more successfully another time. Such a view has, of course, important separatist consequences. The marginal profession is defined in opposition to the core traditions on the margins of which it exists. Marginality, then, becomes defined as an error to be corrected. Opposition by the medical profession is seen as an expression of fear and jealousy, not as an impersonal judgment of objective differences between its own and the marginal practitioner's activities.

FOLK MEDICINE

To understand modern society is to understand the tension between traditional patterns and self-conscious, rational calculations devoted to the mastery of everyday life. To be sure, these contraries involve each other: science is the very essence of a wish for certain knowledge, based on impersonal methods of inquiry leading to shared results open to correction, and intended to replace the claims or revelations of tradition. Yet it should not be forgotten that science can itself grow only within a tradition and within a professional or academic

107

community, and that the exercise of reason, especially in its deductive form, flourished precisely when science existed only intermittently, in the Middle Ages.

The best metaphor for this broad direction of overall change is the spiral. Part of the spring of this spiral comes from the tension between the professions and the laity. In a complex society many people are members of both these spheres, but in different ways. Physicians are the lawyers' clients just as engineers are the doctors' patients. The knowledge of the laity when they turn to medicine, however, unlike that of the laity in need of legal advice, overlaps with the expertise of its potential helpers; no other pairing of the knowledgeable, schooled, expert, or licensed on the one hand, and the half-knowing, uninstructed, inexpert, and unlicensed on the other shows so little contrast.

In spite of its sophisticated laity, however, the medical domain is not likely to be visited by a revolt against the professional healer, as Protestantism revolted against the professional religiouses, and sought to substitute the priesthood of all believers for the occupants of special religious offices. Our standards of health obviously require expertise and specialization; the present distinction between the laity and the professional medical practitioner will disappear only in the unlikely event that we would either come to hold life to be thoroughly cheap and expendable, discounting pain and debility into the bargain, or would radically turn against our whole intellectual history and substitute for it some inclusive idealistic or spiritual alternative. Even if we could choose this latter alternative, the distinctions among the specialist, that is, the specially trained and fully occupied expert, the self-appointed person of special gifts, and the "ordinary" majority would remain. These distinctions inhere in all viable social arrangements that are designed to cope with the full range of exigencies in the lives of individuals.

Cure Beyond the Medical Domain

The contrast between the professional person and the layman is partly a matter of unequal authority. The greater authority of the expert is based on specialized knowledge and competence rather than on special qualities monopolized by some supernaturally favored few. It is no accident, however, that healing has in fact been associated precisely with the special qualities of people who, in their eyes or those of others, are naturally possessed of a more than ordinary power.

The persistence and identity of the medical domain in its professional form and autonomy is assured not only by its contrast with the laity, but also by its organized character. This does not mean that the medical domain cannot become aligned, in varying degrees of intimacy, with other domains of a society, as it has in Russia. Such an alignment, however, exists not for technical purposes, but to combine the bureaucratic patterns of government (or of other large- or small-scale corporate enterprises) with the medical enterprise for the sake of implementing certain ideals of rationality, economy, justice, or control. Ultimately, the medical domain, whatever its degree of autonomy, cannot, as we have seen, monopolize healing. In fact, it does not want to do so, for its task would then be quite out of its reach.

Ailments, illnesses, and debilities, acute or chronic, are obviously of unequal seriousness. Many of them heal themselves. A few are hopeless and must just be borne. These facts define the conditions under which we feel it incumbent to call in a doctor or to go to one. Broadly, all of Western society shares the same standards in this regard, although there are significant variations, both social and idiosyncratic. Although some people hate doctors while others turn to them at the slightest discomfort, all of us in modern societies must practice a fair amount of self-administered medicine. In this we are abetted by a huge flood of public discussion, that is, sustained by our general concern with health. This concern with health yields nonprofessional practices marked by at least a degree of enlightened common sense. Self-administered medicine is part of folk medicine, which can have great variations in sophistication. Folk traditions concerning diagnosis, cure, and prevention of bodily or mental ills thus come to form a halo around a body of professional practices.

Nonprofessional practices naturally include a varied pattern of diagnostic or curative devices. They can include specific prescriptions to prevent pain or palliate it; specific panacean resources such as liquids, herbs, and baths; or acceptance of simplistic theories of the requirements of the human body and the causes of its ill-being.

A few details from the healing ways of the Spanish-speaking peoples of the American Southwest illustrate these points.[2] The ideas of these people are probably derived from four different sources: folk medieval medical lore of Spain, elaborated during several centuries of relative isolation; North American Indian traditions; "Anglo" folk medicine; and "scientific" medical sources. In any specific situation, one or more of these sources might be employed. A given individual can, then, combine a belief in witchcraft or magic with acceptance of some of the medical notions of urban North America.

Mexican folk medicine tends to apply the distinction of hot and cold both to diseases and to cures, and this distinction bears no simple relation to the presence or absence of fever. Cure, rather, consists in the restoration of a balance. (The Hippocratic tradition, as we have noted, was guided by a similar conviction.) Hot diseases are treated with cold remedies, and vice versa, although localities vary in their application of this distinction. In addition to a correct balance of temperature, a clean stomach is an important concern, and health requires the periodic purging of the stomach and of the

[2] L. Saunders, "Healing Ways in the Spanish Southwest," in Jaco, *Patients, Physicians, and Illness,* pp. 189–206.

intestinal tract. Similarly, the blood is important in the maintenance of the state of balance necessary for health: to lose blood is to become weak, even if the loss is small, such as when blood is required for a laboratory test. Such loss of strength is believed to express itself sexually. When men lose blood, they fear the impairment of their sexual vigor.

Illness is conceived primarily in terms of not feeling well. In the absence of subjective feelings of discomfort one is not really ill and has no obligation to do anything about his health. Clearly, our notions about periodic physical check-ups could hardly thrive under Mexican conditions, where people must usually be seriously ill before they begin to seek or accept professional help. There is, even, a tendency to conceal illness, for to be sick is considered a sign of weakness.

Notions of etiology in Mexican folk medicine have room for three kinds of cause: natural, magical, and human. The air, for example, which is a natural element, is intrinsically dangerous, especially at night. Magic includes the power of the evil eye. Within the realm of human motives, strong feelings, including severe frights, can cause illness. When one suffers from magical and human disturbances, a folk specialist, rather than a professional physician, is likely to be called. Because the list of natural diseases is long, so is the range of available remedies.

Spanish-American traditional folk medicine embodies a wide range of curing techniques. These include the use of herbs (Osha, a form of parsley, is one of the most widely used), massages, poultices and plasters, salves, special foods, various types of bathing, prayers, spells, charms, incantations, and, more recently, injections. In some illnesses, several or even all of these techniques are used.

Pregnant women among the Spanish-Americans seldom consult a physician, but carry on as usual, with the addition of a few special precautions. Thus, they avoid the moon-

Health and Healing

light in bed, and if there is an eclipse, they hang keys on a string around their waists lest the baby be deformed by the effect of the moon's shadow falling on them. A mother is advised to have regular bowel movements for some months before her confinement, with the help of castor oil if necessary. When the first movements of the baby are felt, the mother begins to wear a cord or cloth band wrapped tightly around her waist so as to keep the fetus in place and prevent it from damaging her upper organs. Nine days before the expected day of confinement, a series of prayers is begun. Finally, a woman in labor is not permitted to go to bed until after the child is born, but must keep moving, in order to speed up labor.

As this kind of folk knowledge is widely disseminated, anyone giving medical care is subject to the critical attention of the patient's relatives and friends, who are usually ready to insist on changes in treatment or additions to it. Both patient and family, for all their relatively passive attitude to illness, are much more active participants in its cure than are Westerners, who are committed to the mastery of illness. "Anglo" or scientific medicine tends to be regarded as a last resort, to be used only in very serious cases. In this way, modern medicine can hardly achieve a record of impressive success, and thus, by its failures, helps to sustain traditional patterns.

Such traditional patterns are to some extent in the hands of specialists, who are credited with greater than usual knowledge, and who perform special functions. Actually, they work less as individual specialists than as consultants and technicians implementing the therapeutic plans of the patient and his family. These specialists are midwives, general curers, masters of the benevolent and malevolent techniques implied by witchcraft, and thwarters of evil powers. All these practitioners are paid in goods or cash for their services. In most instances, however, the commercial part of the transaction is said to be subordinate to its therapeutic intent.

"Anglo" scientific medicine is carried on in the context of rather impersonal relations between doctors and patients, and it often involves procedures that lie beyond the ken of its beneficiaries. Patients, moreover, are treated one at a time; their relatives are not to interfere; they are to cooperate with a variety of authorities, including doctors and nurses, and they must pay handsomely for treatment. Folk medicine, on the other hand, allows for personal relations, is executed through familiar procedures, and is compatible with active participation by the patient and his family. Folk medicine can take place at home, is much less expensive than "Anglo" medicine, and it leaves control over the situation in the hands of the patient and those he trusts.

This is a condensed and oversimplified account that is not meant to suggest that folk-medicine is a matter of native traditions alone. Urban and industrial populations also participate in medical traditions that contrast with accepted professional practice. The halo of marginal medicine that surrounds the medical core will probably always be itself encircled by a still wider halo of folk practices.

QUACKERY

I have argued that cure can never be a monopoly. It will always be practiced, especially on minor ailments, without the assistance of professional help. Moreover, given our activist preferences, what is officially defined as incurable or hopeless will not always be passively accepted as such by the victims of the debility. This situation provides an opportunity for quacks. Unlike malpractitioners and marginal practitioners, who are confined to the ranks of the licensed, quacks are practitioners who are neither licensed nor competent. They misrepresent the physical conditions of their patients and the diagnostic or curative efficacy of their methods of treatment. They also misrepresent their own education and skill. In general, their activities accrue to the physical detriment or financial loss of those who seek their help. Perhaps quacks represent a proportion of any community's quota of knaves. Presumably quacks, unlike marginal practitioners, are motivated by financial gain rather than by faith in alternative solutions to problems and plights.

We know from a California study[3] that quackery is subject to the provisions of those codes that govern the licensing of businesses and professions, of health and safety, especially through the agency of the Pure Food and Drugs Act, and through the Penal Code. In addition to being a kind of spurious medical practice, quackery can be considered a form of theft or conspiracy. In spite of this illegal tinge, however, comprehensive legislation to deal effectively with medical quackery is difficult to obtain. Zeal for the protection of health and the punishment of crime must be balanced against the right of an individual to make his living, a customer to choose among alternative services, and the unorthodox to experiment.

To some extent quackery is a specialized matter, with the specialty changing through time. For some time it tended to be concentrated on the treatment of cancer. It may well be that as quackery regarding cancer cures is diminished, it will instead turn up in connection with heart disease or schizophrenia or tuberculosis.

There is a form of nonlicensed practicing of professional activities that is nevertheless not real quackery, as when people practice ordinary medicine in the absence of actual training for it and are not discovered for some considerable time. Similarly, there exist fraudulent priests or lawyers, practicing within the professional domain and misrepresenting their

[3] "Quackery in California," *Stanford Law Review,* 1959, 2(2), pp. 265–296.

identity, but not defying the traditions of the profession they simulate. Sociologically, the difference between those who indulge in quackery knowingly and, hence, primarily for money, and those who indulge in it in good faith bears scrutiny, because it represents the grey area between the downright fraudulent and the merely misguided. It is difficult to know how much quackery occurs; it is relatively easy to speculate, as we have done, as to why it exists at all. The wish for swift solutions to problems, ignorance of the dangers of quackery, fear of doctors, and perhaps the wish to protect the respectable and professional resources of our society, all these surely combine to ensure quackery some continued existence.

Quacks are to be clearly distinguished from those marginal practitioners who practice alternatives to medical care, such as chiropractors and Christian Scientists. Unlike quacks, these practitioners are not involved in mispresentation, but are guided by a specific theory of illness. For Christian Scientists, for example, the cause of disturbances is taken to be a foregone conclusion, and diagnosis and treatment are self-evidently contained in the body of teaching that constitutes their theory and approach.

To oversimplify, one may think of Christian Science as a form of radical idealism because it contends that only mind exists. Evil, sin, disease, and death are linked with one another and with matter. Such feelings are, therefore, unreal. To believe in them is to commit an error, and to indulge the illusions of the mortal mind. Sickness, as an erroneous belief, will cease when the mind disabuses itself of its error. Healing, therefore, must literally consist in arguing down false beliefs and in convincing the patient that his sickness is not real and persuading him that he is quite well. The healer makes no diagnosis and need not be present in person, but can have an effect at a distance. Medical science, from this point of view, becomes a rather extensive fabric of make-believe. Its success must in the main be attributed, from the Christian Science point of view, to the patient's faith in his doctor.

Clearly such a position raises a number of problems because it can obviously not be consistently carried out. Christian Science readers do, on the one hand, wear glasses, but, on the other hand, they can place in danger those who do not share their belief but are nevertheless associated with them or exposed to them. As a religious movement Christian Science reminds the medical profession of the importance of nonrational elements both in the genesis and the restitution of sickness. As an activity carried out in good faith, involving no financial gain or misrepresentation, it cannot be written off as quackery. We might perhaps think of it as an instance of medical sectarianism, as well as a form of faith healing. It rejects contemporary medical practice, not because of ignorance, but because of its commitment to a radically different theological or philosophical assumption.

It is one of the marks of Western society to make such differences possible. This leads to a variety of conflicts and issues, whose resolution demands rather delicate compromises. A radical prohibition of quackery would in its course suppress Christian Science or other healing cults, and such a suppression would constitute a serious infringement of personal liberty. On the other hand, complete indifference to the existence of marginal practitioners and quacks would expose nonbelievers, who are themselves exposed to believers, to hazards of health from which they have a right to be protected. All of these things illustrate once again that health and illness are inevitably both an individual and a public matter, and suggest some reasons for our persistent concern with it.

Index

A

Accidents, 11
Accreditation of medical education, 66
Activism: effects of, 2–3; and pain, 43; religious support for, 8. *See also* Mastery
Administration and medical domain, 61
Africa, medical manpower in, 11
Alcoholism, 13; causes of, 14–15; among Jews and Irish, 14; meaning of, 16
Allocation of medical resources, 99
American Medical Association, 20, 21, 22
ANDERSON, O. W., 86, 96
ANSHEN, R., 27
Appendicitis, 31
ARENDT, H., 42
ASCLEPIUS, 7–8
Attitudes: of medical profession, 19; toward mental illness, 38. *See also* Medical practice
Autonomy: of the body, 31; medical, 52–54

B

BECKER, H. S., 66, 70
Body, implications of for medical practice, 24–32
Body image: and illness, 30; and pain, 42; source of, 26
British Health Service, 22, 87, 96, 99

British Medical Association, 22
Bureaucracy: and medical education, 65; and medical practice, 96–97

C

Canadian hospital insurance, 99
Cancer, 10, 11, 13
Careers: education for medical, 64–69; for married women, 23; medical, 62; medical vs. nursing, 65; nursing, 71
CARPER, J. W., 66
Childbirth: in Mexico, 110–113; and pain, 47
Chiropractors, 13; compared with medical doctors, 102–105
Choice of physician: general discussion of, 75–79; as myth, 88
Christian Science, 5–6, 7, 102; defined, 115–116
Clergymen: as counselors, 33; compared with doctors, 17, 59
Clinical encounters, characteristics of, 80–84. *See also* Doctor-patient relationship
Clinical practice. *See* Medical practice
Commitment in medicine, 70
Common sense and health practices, 110
Continuity of care, 64
Contract: in clinical encounter, 81; in doctor-patient relationship, 75, 99
Cost: of illness, 9; of medical care, 87–100; of medical schools,

117

Index

94; of specialization, 63. *See also* Fees
Crime, 39
Culture and expression of pain, 44–46
CUMMING, E., 39
CUMMING, J., 39
Cure, nonmedical, 101–102

D

Death, 26; and dying, 47–49
Degenerative disease, 10
Delinquency, 39
Deliria, 35
Depression, 35
Dermatology, 59
DEUTSCHER, I., 71
Developing countries and communicable diseases, 10
Differentiation and administration, 61. *See also* Division of Labor; Specialization
Dilettantism as specialization, 60
Discipline in clinical encounter, 84
Division of labor: as differentiation, 53, 61; in medical domain, 58; in medicine and education, 55; in medicine and religion, 54. *See also* Specialization
Doctor-patient relationship: asymmetry in, 81, 94; as contract, 99; discussed, 74; and expectations, 22; and fees, 95–96; in folk vs. Anglo medicine, 113; as red herring, 88; and trust, 75

E

ECKSTEIN, H., 87, 96
Economy of health, 4. *See also* Costs
Eczema, 31
Education: in medical schools, 12, 94; as profession, 55. *See also* Medical students

Egalitarianism and health, 4
Ego, Freudian view of, 36
Emotional disturbances, 13
Engineering, compared with medicine, 17
Epilepsy, 34–35
Equality of medical care, 21; as a value, 4, 7
ERICKSON, E., 80, 81
Ethics, professional, 17
Ethnicity and physician choice, 78
Europe, medical manpower in, 12

F

Faith healing, 182
Family doctor: compared with chiropractor, 106; as coordinator, 61; as general practitioner, 62–63; respect for, 63
Fear, 6
Fees: and doctor-patient relationship, 81; effect of on practice, 95–97. *See also* Cost
FEIN, R., 90
FIELD, M. G., 97
Financial arrangements of physicians, 92. *See also* Cost; Fees
Fluoridation, 7
Folk medicine, 102; in Mexico, 107–113; and professionalization, 56
FOX, R., 68–69
Freedom: and cost of care, 91; and illness, 16
FREUD, S., 99; view of man of, 35–36
FROMM, E., 27
Fun, as value, 2–3

G

GEER, B., 66, 70
General practitioner, 62–63. *See also* Family doctor
GLAD, D. D., 14

118

Index

Medical autonomy, 52, 54; and method of payment, 97
Medical colleagueship, 20–21
Medical costs. *See* Costs
Medical debts, 98
Medical domain: general discussion of, 50–61; and other institutions, 109; rejection of, 7. *See also* Medical profession; Medical practice
Medical education, general discussion of, 64–69. *See also* Medical students
Medical journals, 21
Medical knowledge, 56, 60. *See also* Science and medicine; Medical education; Tensions, intellectual
Medical licensing, 21
Medical offenses, 21
Medical organizations, 20–22
Medical practice: clinical, 55; as fiduciary relationship, 81; general discussion of, 96–97. *See also* Medical domain; Professions; Tensions, social
Medical profession: and the body, 29; commitment to, 70; international character of, 56; and mental illness, 33. *See also* Professions; Medical domain; Medical practice
Medical research, 62
Medical resources, allocation of, 99
Medical schools, 12, 94. *See also* Medical education
Medical specialization. *See* Specialization
Medical students: careers of, 62; role of, 72; self-image of, 71
Medical teaching, 62. *See also* Medical education
Medical tradition, 21, 51–53, 58–59

Medicine as occupation, 19. *See also* Careers
Melancholia, 35
Mental illness, 11; general discussion of, 32–41. *See also* Illness; Pain; Suffering; Tensions, social
MERTON, R. K., 62, 66, 72
Mexican folk medicine, 110–113
Mind: and body, 24–32; illness of, 32–41
Moral neutrality in medicine, 54–55
Moral problem in mental illness, 34
Mourning, 48

N

National Chiropractic Association, 103
National Institute of Health, 98
Nearsightedness, 31
Negro doctors, 79
Neurotics, 104
Nonmedical aspects of medicine, 102
Nonmedical cure, 101
Nonprofessional practice, 109–110
"Normal," distinguished from abnormal, 37
Nursing, as career, 71

O

Office visits, cost of, 86
Old Americans and pain, 44–46
Organizational context of health, 6
Organizations, professional, 16, 20–22
Orthodontics as specialty, 59–60

P

Pain: and cost, 93; general discussion of, 24–52; as punishment, 3; and religion, 8–9. *See also* Suffering; Illness
Paranoia, 35
Parasitic diseases, 10

Index

Index

SNYDER, C. R., 14

Social class and physician choice, 78

Socialization: to medicine, 64; of patients, 19

Society, effect on illness and health, 5, 15, 99; effect on medical practice, 97, 109; effect on mental illness, 33–38; effect on pain, 44. *See also* Tensions, social

Sociology in medical education, 66

Specialists, coordination of, 60–61. *See also* Specialization

Specialization: general discussion of, 58–64; and medical education, 68; and physician choice, 75; and professionalization, 56; and quackery, 114

Specialties, status of, 63. *See also* Specialization

Standards in medical education, 66

Students, nursing, 68. *See also* Medical students

Suffering: and mental illness, 40; and pain, 42. *See also* Pain; Illness

Surgeons, 63

Surgery, 59

T

TB, 31

Tensions, of doctors: autonomy vs. cooperation with other agents, 52, 55; compassion vs. profit, 18–19, 21, 51; economic vs. social vs. technical aspects of role, 95; freedom vs. constraint in practice, 99–100; need for vs. disapproval of chiropractors, 105; science vs. clinical care, 18–19, 56, 58, 65, 89; specialization vs. well-roundedness, 18–19

Tensions, intellectual: body vs. mind, 32; causal complexity vs. simplicity, 13; experience vs. thought, 24–25; humanism vs. science, 57–58, 106; specialization vs. dilettantism, 60; traditional vs. rational solutions, 107

Tensions, of patients: acceptance vs. mastery of illness, 57; folk vs. professional medicine, 112; freedom of choice vs. quality of care, 89; helplessness vs. attention in illness, 31–32

Tensions, social: Hygeia vs. Asclepius, 7–8; legitimate vs. marginal practice, 106; private vs. public health insurance, 88–89; professionals vs. laity, 108–109; treat mentally ill vs. protect society, 38–39; treat mentally ill vs. redefine "normal," 41

Tradition. *See* Medical tradition

U

Ulcers, 13

United Nations, 10, 11

Urbanization and medical care, 61

V

Values regarding illness and health, 2–9. *See also* Tensions, social

Vegetarian, 7

Veterans Administration, 98

W

WARDWELL, W. I., 103

WARMBRUNN, W., 22

WILLIAMS, J. J., 76, 77, 78

Women physicians, 23, 76–79

World Health Organization, 10

Z

ZBOROWSKI, M., 44

122

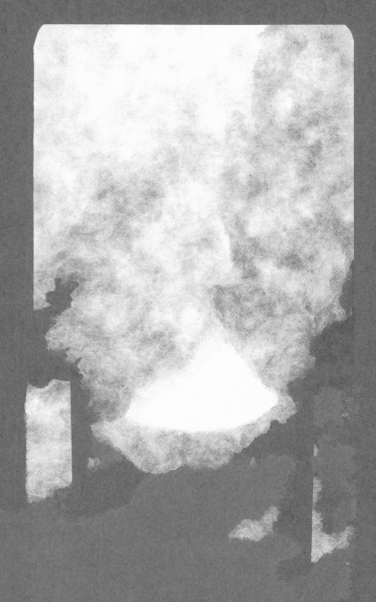